Only Connect

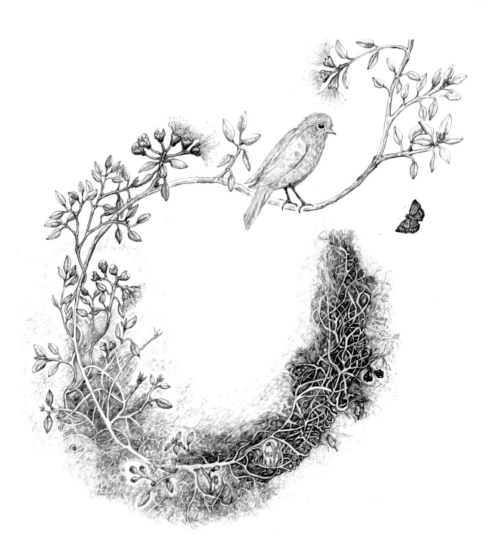

Only Connect

Poems and Stories from
New Zealand Music Therapy

Edited by Claire Molyneux

Foreword by Sarah Hoskyns

Only Connect: Poems and Stories from New Zealand Music Therapy
ISBN 978-0-473-40630-1.

A catalogue record for this book is available from the National Library of New Zealand.

Published by Mountain Girl Publishing, Nelson, New Zealand.
Ph +64 (0) 21 0819 8918.

f Mountain Girl Publishing

First published 2017

Cover art: 'The Songsters' by Anne Bailey.
Cover design by Stephanie Nierstenhoefer.
Illustrations by Robina Adamson.
Design and layout by Chris Rutter.

Published with the assistance of a grant from the Erika Schloss Fund, Music Therapy New Zealand.

All proceeds from the sale of the book are donated to Music Therapy New Zealand.

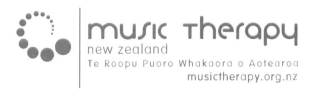

musictherapy.org.nz

*Dedicated to my mother for
bringing music and poetry into my life*

Each of the stories in this book has been shared with permission from the individual or their family members. In some cases, real names have been used at the request of the individual or their family. In other cases, names and some identifying details have been changed to protect their identities.

Contents

III – Personal Journeys

Foreword

Nearly twenty years ago, I was leading a termly meeting on a wintry evening with supervisor colleagues for the music therapy training programme at Guildhall School, London. We were discussing our week-at-work as an opening to the session's agenda. One member of the group described going to a clinical team meeting the previous day to review work with a young child. Shyly she told us that instead of her expected brief prose report, she had stood up and offered a poem. She had felt unable to capture the beauty of a little child's new attempts to walk with the funky and funny songs they had been sharing. So - bravely - in front of the consultant paediatrician, head teacher, therapy team and parents, she had delivered her creative offering. The parents were incredibly touched, several teachers cried, and we as a supervising team were joyful about her bold move. Of course it is not always possible to disrupt the regular clinical meeting process in this way, but what a surprise and pleasure when it happens!

I am delighted and honoured to welcome you to this collection of writings by music therapists from Aotearoa New Zealand celebrating a topic that echoes this event long ago, and very near to my heart; that is, the artistic responsiveness of therapists to their own practice. Claire Molyneux and the New Zealand music therapist authors represented here have created an elegant and refreshing book about people, music, place, time and the music therapy relationships that have evolved. I have taught or worked closely with each of them, and feel proud and excited to observe their creativity. This is a risky old road for people to put themselves on, and to dare, with some different forms and modes of art. And of course this may or may not communicate how they would hope. Such is the uncertainty of the arts. Nevertheless the team of writers have brought much richness to this journey, and I challenge you to *not* be moved and changed by the accounts of beautifully diverse work that are shared in the following pages. The writers have worked often in a different and new way to communicate a truth, a careful thought, a feeling. Words are tricky places and I have had many of my own tearful experiences trying to force meaningful therapeutic moments into the constraints of academic or 'clinical' language and form. Of course creative writing can be just as unforgiving, but I have found artistic integration and life infusing these mini-journeys-of-the-soul here unfolding for the readers of this book.

It is very timely for these stories and poems to be published in Aotearoa in 2017. There is burgeoning interest in creating research in the mode of the art form, as witnessed in the 2015 special edition, volume 52, of the American *Journal of Music Therapy* on arts-based research, and widely varied methodologies explored in the international journal *The Arts in Psychotherapy* (Edwards, 2016). This is added to increasingly strong valuing of the flexible, malleable, communicative nature of *musicians* as core to the identity of music therapy internationally (Kenny, 2015; Viega & Forinash, 2016). Claire Molyneux's insightful and innovative introduction to the collection cites the growing community of practitioners calling upon music therapists to document and share their work using such artful methods.

While we concentrate to 'be there for our participants or clients', music therapists are regularly barometers of the emotional climate in their music therapy settings. I have been charmed to read about the diverse temperatures, feelings, atmospheres and practices that the therapists have captured in their short opening frames about their own music therapy rooms which characterise the book's first section. And we get to know so much more about the diverse music therapy spaces that individual practitioners have created as the book progresses. To me there is something especially honest about this. We don't ever really know how it is for our participants, but can merely read the possibilities, and suggest, through our own responsiveness to our encounters with them. Therefore capturing energetically and imaginatively what each music therapist has made of these moments seems to be such a right and proper thing to do. With judgement, sensitivity and perhaps some luck, it could be shared by our children, adults, and older folk with whom we make a contract.

In the course of creating the poems and stories, the writers have happened upon some ingenious metaphors, touching phrases and funny motifs to capture their meaning. In no particular order, here are some examples:

'In the summer, I open all the windows ... to cool the room down. I close them again before we start, to prevent the smaller instruments ending up in the car park below.'

'Sometimes we settled for songs about the rain and the seagulls that made rhythms on our roof.'

'... fun is baking soda to the human spirit'

'... round the room whizzing whirling here we are in the music room squeezing behind the piano you and me in the music room reappearing hurrying scurrying bounding pounding drumbeats matching footsteps won't stop can't stop after sitting sitting sitting ...'

'... you bit your hand or grabbed my arm, squeezing it hard. We called this dysregulation, but I suspect it was your way of trying to let me know something.'

'"We thought we were here for Ella, but Ella was here for us", your mum explained.'

Fly my creatures, fly to find them in the following pages. Enjoy where they take you. Not a *luxury* nor a diversion (Lorde, 1984), but necessary and inspiring food for thought.

Dr Sarah Hoskyns
NZ RMTh, HCPC(UK) Music Therapist
Victoria University of Wellington, July 2017.

References

Edwards, J. (2016). The breadth and depth of contemporary creative arts therapy publications and research. *The Arts in Psychotherapy, 51*, A1. doi:http://dx.doi.org/10.1016/j.aip.2016.11.001

Kenny, C. (2015). Performing theory: Playing in the music therapy discourse. *Journal of Music Therapy, 52*(4), 457-486. doi:10.1093/jmt/thv019

Lorde, A. (1984). Poetry is not a luxury. In *Sister outsider: Poems and speeches by Audre Lorde*. New York: The Crossing Press.

Viega, M., & Forinash, M. (2016). Arts-based research. In B. Wheeler & K. Murphy (Eds.), *Music Therapy Research* (pp. 491-504). Dallas TX, USA: Barcelona Publishers.

Introduction

Claire Molyneux

Connecting with music therapy writing

An encounter in the music therapy room exists beyond, within and without words and yet our efforts to communicate what takes place are often reduced to words. The question of how we communicate the dance between those in the therapy room has preoccupied music therapists and led to much philosophical and theoretical debate. This collection of writing does not attempt to add to that debate but simply to share the poetry of our encounters in the therapy room, responding to the call by music therapist, Mary Rykov, 'for even more poetry-centred accounts because writing is such a crucial competency for communicating about music therapy research and practice' (2011, p.6).

In my professional life as a music therapist, I have always been aware of the efforts to distill the essence of the complex therapeutic encounter into prose including narrative reports, goals and focus areas and summaries of progress. And yet I know that no written report can fully convey the experience in the therapy room; the complexity and frailty of human nature, the strength and fragility of human relationships and the loneliness inherent in the search for a shared moment of connectedness. The goals, focus areas and written reports are a tool that show only part of the encounter. In an effort to communicate to others there are times I have self-consciously offered a poem or piece of expressive prose to accompany a report with the goal of conveying the ineffable and intangible aspects of the work. Our efforts to capture what transpired or emerged in a therapy session are frequently frustrated as the process of writing or speaking about the encounter transforms it, only revealing partial knowings, never the whole.

This collection of writing is about love, values and journeys. It was born out of my personal preoccupation with balancing the demand for objective evidence with the poesis of the therapeutic endeavour. On unpacking my belongings recently after moving from New Zealand back to England, I looked again at my first music therapy essays written in training more than 20 years ago. Nearly all of them started with a quote from a literary source; poetry or prose. In the early part of my professional life I felt it necessary to weed this desire for poetry out of my writing; it wasn't academic or scholarly enough, not objective. However, embraced by the rich culture and landscape of New Zealand, I began, in turn, to embrace my need for an artistic and creative telling of my music therapy practice and to seek ways to share this with others.

The recent interest in arts-based research, poetry and vocative texts used in music therapy research to both analyse, present and disseminate data is encouraging (Arnason & Seabrook, 2010; Jessop, 2014; Ledger & McCaffrey, 2015; Ledger & Edwards, 2011; Nicol, 2008). Although this book doesn't seek to add to academic debate, I acknowledge the helpful literature that discusses the value of creatively writing our work. Music therapist Carolyn Arnason reflects on writing as 'a refuge in the often confusing land of qualitative research' (2010, p.2), and, together with Seabrook, discusses the value of creative writing to assist with the processes of reflection, synthesis and understanding. Seabrook states: 'For me, an arts-based understanding of a phenomenon is akin to a most beautiful arts-based understanding of life; it offers few concrete answers, rather a blossoming of the self that allows an opening up to new and richer understandings' (p.15). Jessop's research (2014) 'used poetry, metaphor, and imagery to represent participants in a dementia care music therapy group, highlighting their humanity, their musicality, and ultimately their experiences of musical self-actualization' (p.49). Jessop argues that the rationale for using creative means to present research findings and participants is 'to better represent the human quality of lived experience and to more fully engage readers holistically, emotionally, intellectually, and viscerally' (p.51).

The valuable contribution that arts-based research can make to music therapy is discussed by Ledger and McCaffrey (2015) and Ledger and Edwards (2011) who encourage music therapists to enter 'this new terrain' which can 'develop compelling findings, to deepen understandings of their research materials, and to promote dialogue and reflection' (p.317). They describe the challenges to music therapists of describing research as 'artistic' due to the dominant discourse in healthcare which requires 'evidence' within a positivist frame (p.315). Furthermore, Ledger and Edwards acknowledge the personal challenge for music therapists sharing their work in more intimate and artistic ways; that although the poetry or creative writing emerges from the therapeutic process, we may worry that it is not of 'sufficient critical standard' and may feel embarrassed to share our writing with others (p.315). I am deeply indebted to the writers and therapists who have contributed to this book, who confidently show some of themselves on the page. Each piece of writing has been carefully crafted, building on the lived experience in the therapy room, with authors using as a starting point the clinical notes and recordings of sessions in the context of their own observations and experience. Creatively writing our work as music therapists can help to process and understand the embodied and embedded experiences of working nonverbally and verbally in a finely attuned way. This idea is supported by current research being undertaken by PhD candidate and New Zealand Registered Music Therapist Carolyn Ayson. Using an arts-based auto-ethnographic approach for her research titled *An autoethnography of a practitioner-patient: Exploring the counterpoint* (working title), Ayson stated 'The use of more poetic language is needed at times as language devoid of emotion and imagination cannot support this body of mine and the experiences I have had' (2016). Furthermore, poetic anthropologist and autoethnographer, Ruth Behar, states that her work as a poetic anthropologist allowed her 'to experience the emotionally wrenching ways in which we attain knowledge of others and ourselves' (2008, p.63).

Rykov (2007) supports the inclusion of different ways of writing and presenting music therapy work, suggesting that the disruption of conventional discursive research and representation can expand 'the realm of searching, re-searching, asking, telling, knowing and showing' (p.379). Rykov further develops this argument in her 2011 essay in which she states her goal 'is to illustrate and inspire writing about music therapy that is creative and nondiscursive. Such writing occurs by listening intently, contemplating, and responding' (p.1). She has also noted the connection that creative writing fosters with the real encounters and experiences therapists have:

> Striving for poetry while remaining close to the essence of music therapy experience is not self-indulgent gazing reserved for reflexive journals only. We need to strive for poetry because the scientific ideal of objectivity veers us away from lived reality. We need poetic method to bring us closer to knowing and communicating the essence of being, particularly for instances of nonverbal, embodied experience such as music and music therapy (p.7).

The poems and stories in this book build on the invitation to present the complexities of the music therapy relationship in creative ways. The aim is to experientially engage the reader; to have impact, create connections and resonances, invite sensory responses and dialogue. As Pavlicevic puts it, 'The richer and more complex our understandings and insights, the richer the experiences we are able to share with clients' (1999, p. 142).

Connecting with the New Zealand music therapy community

Several years ago I wrote and submitted to the New Zealand Journal of Music Therapy a first draft of the story *Only Connect,* knowing it was unlikely to be accepted as it was not written in an academic style. I did however get a positive response from the then Editor, Karen Twyford, who suggested it might be developed into an idea for a book. Some years later, I put out a call for expressions of interest to New Zealand music therapists to contribute writing that subjectively described the lived experience of music therapy in a way that celebrated the poetic and lyrical nature of the work. I had a vision that a book could capture the more private and personal writing with which music therapists might engage to help understand and process their experiences. A number of therapists committed to writing for the book and a process of co-editing commenced. The authors were invited to write creatively about an experience that moved them; writing was framed as a form of personal freedom, a way to understand experience. About half of the group of writers attended a writing retreat at the beautiful Teal Bay in the Bay of Islands, New Zealand. This retreat helped us to connect in a way that supported the sharing of our stories and enthusiasm for writing our therapeutic encounters, with lively discussion that helped identify commonalities and differences. Further editing and re-writing took place as the structure, form and content of the book began to be realised. This emphasis on collaboration has been essential to the project and reflects something of my experience of music therapy in Aotearoa New Zealand. Although all of the pieces in the book are written by single authors, the power of collaboration and the collective voice has been a strong influence. The stories reflect a desire to re-position music therapy writing outside a particular approach, academic language or workplace structure, seeking the freedom to write in a way that speaks more closely to the experience of practice.

Connecting with the New Zealand context

New Zealand (NZ) music therapy has grown rapidly, 'from 36 Registered Music Therapists in 2008 to 75 in 2016' (Molyneux, Talmage & McGann, 2016). NZ music therapists are actively engaged in research alongside a growing body of master's level research by music therapy students. A few recent publications show the range of research areas including professional identity (Warren & Rickson, 2016), music therapy and autism (Rickson, Castelino, Molyneux, Ridley & Upjohn-Beatson, 2016; Rickson, Molyneux, Ridley, Castelino & Upjohn-Beatson, 2015), community music therapy (Rickson & Skewes McFerran, 2014), neurological choirs (Talmage, Ludlam, Leão, Fogg & Purdy, 2013), special education (Twyford, 2013), and practice and research in training (Hoskyns, 2014, 2011). NZ music therapists have published their work widely in journals and books in the fields of music therapy and health. There is considerable effort directed towards creating a strong and clear evidence base for the benefits of music therapy supported by the charitable work of Music Therapy New Zealand who, as well as promoting and increasing awareness, provide grants to establish new projects and research activities. As a small community of professionals, NZ music therapists strive to increase their presence in the international community through research, presentations and musical contributions such as the World Federation of Music Therapy 30th Anniversary songwriting competition which was jointly won by NZ Music Therapist Ahjay Stelino (aka Ajay Castelino). The development of music therapy in NZ has been ably documented by Croxson (2001, 2003, 2007) and Fletcher (2016) along with the significant role played by the Raukatauri Music Therapy Centre acknowledged by Molyneux (2013).

This collection of writing is grounded in the practice of therapists living and working in New Zealand, alongside a background of academic and clinical achievements. Each writer embodies something of their own interconnectedness and immersion in the culture of this unique country and community of therapists. This process echoes Kenny's call that 'each country must take the responsibility to create a unique expression of beauty and all its variations within a culture, as these will have a direct relationship to the success of music therapy practice in each region' (2006, p.181). Furthermore, the enthusiasm and commitment of the contributors to this project demonstrates a desire in New Zealand for a different kind of writing about the experience of music therapy.

The cover artwork and illustrations have been chosen specifically to ground the writing in the landscape of Aotearoa New Zealand. From a personal perspective, the natural world, the song of native birds, the ebb and flow of the seasons have been central to my experience and relationship with Aotearoa. Moreover, the physical environment and our relationship to it is held centrally within Māori models of health such as Te Whare Tapa Whā (Durie, 1998) and Te Wheke (Pere, 1997) which illustrate the interdependence and connectedness of all things physical and spiritual. 'Traditional Māori health acknowledges the link between the mind, the spirit, the human connection with whānau, and the physical world in a way that is seamless and uncontrived. Until the introduction of Western medicine there was no division between them' (Ministry of Health, 2017). There is a growing dialogue between NZ music therapists and Māori traditional healers and musicians which brings new understandings of the ways in which sound and song connect with the physical world, health and medicine (Rollo, 2013; Fletcher, DeAth Green, MacDonald & Hoskyns, 2014, Hoskyns & Roestenburg, in press). The process of partnership is the theme of the recent publication *Collaborative and indigenous mental health therapy: Tātaihono – Stories of Māori healing and psychiatry* (NiaNia, Bush & Epston, 2017) which explores the relationship between psychiatry and traditional healing within a Māori mental health service.

The illustrations in the book are by Robina Adamson who describes her connection with birdsong, music and the natural world:

> When I was around seven years old, I was just recovering from whooping cough which had left me very weak, and needing one year off school to convalesce. I then had a serious fall and a head

injury. I didn't speak for a long time, had short term memory loss and terrible headaches. I believe a thrush that sang in a tree outside our dining room window helped with my healing. I couldn't speak as I didn't seem to remember words. I couldn't retrieve them in my mind, or create a spoken word. When I tried, the pain in my head became overwhelming. Somehow the bird song didn't do that, and seemed to me at the time to be a language outside spoken speech and that communication was clearer and more real to me than my family in the room trying to talk to me. That is why I relate music and healing to birdsong so strongly, and felt drawn to include birds in the artwork.

The illustrations depict a range of native and introduced flora and fauna including tiny manuka flowers which are not only beautiful but have healing qualities. The violets represent springtime and new beginnings and connect with Mali, Robina's daughter, the young woman who was the inspiration for *Only Connect*; the deep purple being one of her favourite colours. The three little birds are New Zealand Welcome Swallow babies sitting on the branch of a kowhai tree. The lady bug is on its own journey surrounded by tiny life forms of lichen. The frontispiece depicts a spiral of growth and change and is described by Robina:

The right side is the beginning and the circle moves clockwise. At the beginning it looks dead, like bones, desolate. As I drew the darkest parts at the right side of the circle, I kept thinking that even in the darkest parts of everything there is always light. We don't always notice it at first, but to me that is the magic, hope, spirit, or whatever you perceive it to be, of life. You will see those tiny specks of light dancing about in the picture. It is one of those specks that has settled into a dark pocket, and from that little sparkle, hope grows. The first snowdrop emerges, then another. Leaves and new buds on the pohutukawa structure appear, then you will see a change in direction in the main support of everything. Small leaves and flowers appear and become progressively stronger and bigger, then the North Island Robin appears in the sunlight near the top but still with scope for more journey yet to come. The tiny butterfly is an endangered native species called Coastal Copper. It is a lovely orange with black markings and extremely small. The little robin is symbolic of the journey a person might make in therapy as they emerge further into the sunlight and wider world connected through the music. The butterfly represents the world around and evokes the curiosity of the robin.

The cover art is by Anne Bailey, former Director of the Raukatauri Music Therapy Centre (2008-2012) and now full-time artist. It is called *The Songsters* and shows the Shining Cuckoo, Grey Warbler and Tui, all who have distinctive voices.

Connection: Final thoughts

Reading the writing of others has been a way I have sought connection. As an adolescent, I immersed myself in the writing of poets such as Maya Angelou, Emily Dickinson, A. S. J. Tessimond, Ted Hughes and T. S Eliot. Later, reading bel hooks and finding my way to Paulo Freire and Audre Lorde, discovering New Zealand poets Glenn Colquhoun and Dinah Hawken, I am convinced of the necessity of sharing stories from music therapy in creative forms. This ability to connect powerfully with self and others through creative writing is highlighted in Audre Lorde's compelling essay *Poetry is not a luxury* (1984) which positions poetry as a tool for activism and revolution. There is some of that spirit in this book too, although from a different context and time. Carolyn Kenny (2006), discussing the place of beauty in music therapy practice and the role of engagement in the arts for both client and therapist, offers examples of poems written following sessions with patients. She suggests that this continuance of the 'aesthetic interplay' between therapist and patient helps deepen our understanding and experience of the work of therapy through acknowledgement of the beauty inherent in being human and finding ways to be human together.

This collection of writing is organised into three parts. The first section consists of a series of descriptions of therapy rooms. The setting in which music therapists work varies enormously. One thing that is striking about these pieces of writing is the way in which the therapists carefully consider the instruments and environment, preparing the rooms to facilitate the therapeutic journey for each client or group of clients. The middle section offers a selection of poems and stories from music therapy practice across the lifespan. The final section presents four pieces of writing that explore the more personal journey of the music therapist, addressing issues of professional and cultural identity, alongside the process of discovery and growth that comes with training and practice. The writers and I acknowledge the individuals and families who have generously given consent for their stories to be published. In some cases, real names have been used at the request of the individual or family and in others, names and some identifying details have been changed to protect confidentiality. In all cases a process of gaining informed consent has been carefully followed.

As this book seeks connection, I would like to finish this introduction by turing briefly to the choice of title. The words *Only Connect* come from Howards End by E. M. Forster: 'Only connect! That was the whole of her sermon. Only connect the prose and the passion, and both will be exalted, and human love will be seen at its highest. Live in fragments no longer. Only connect, and the beast and the monk, robbed of the isolation that is life to either, will die' (2000, p.159). For me, the process of writing about music therapy is all about connection: to connect the poetry and the prose with the endeavour to understand and gain insight; to connect the lyrical process inherent in both the music therapy session and our description of it; and to connect the experience of being with and being without. The stories offered in this book are not truths, but expressions of lived experiences; frames and snapshots into a private world that both contain and omit. As Jeanette Winterson (2011) puts it:

> Truth for anyone is a very complex thing. For a writer, what you leave out says as much as those things you include. What lies beyond the margin of the text? The photographer frames the shot; writers frame their world ...
>
> When we tell a story we exercise control, but in such a way as to leave a gap, an opening. It is a version, but never the final one. And perhaps we hope that the silences will be heard by someone else, and the story can continue, can be retold.
>
> When we write we offer the silence as much as the story. Words are the part of silence that can be spoken (p.8).

With that thought, I leave you to read and connect with the words and silences of the stories that follow.

References

Arnason, C., & Seabrook, D. (2010). Reflections on change in arts-based research: The experience of two music therapists. *Voices: A World Forum For Music Therapy, 10*(1). doi:10.15845/voices.v10i1.154

Ayson, C. (2016). *Seeing the unseen: A post-structural look at disability in music therapy.* Music Therapy New Zealand Hui, Auckland, New Zealand, August 2016.

Behar, R. (2008). Between poetry and anthropology: Searching for languages of home. In M. Cahnmann-Taylor & R. Siegesmund (Eds.). *Arts-based research in education* (pp.55-71). New York: Routledge.

Croxson, M. (2001). New Zealand and music therapy: A synopsis of a new scene. *Voices: A World Forum For Music Therapy, 1*(1). doi:10.15845/voices.v1i1.41

Croxson, M. (2003). Music therapy in New Zealand. *Voices Resources.* Retrieved January 08, 2015, from http://testvoices.uib.no/community/?q=country/monthnewzealand_february2003

Croxson, M. (2007). Music therapy in New Zealand. *Voices Resources.* Retrieved January 10, 2015, from http://testvoices.uib.no/community/?q=country/monthnewzealand_april2007

Durie, M. H. (1998). *Whaiora: Māori health development* (2nd Edition). Oxford University Press.

Fletcher, H., DeAth Green, C., MacDonald, M., & Hoskyns, S. (2014). Rāranga wairua: Creative cultural collaboration in an infant child and adolescent mental health service. *New Zealand Journal of Music Therapy 12*: 87-105.

Fletcher, H. (2016). Invited essay: A brief history of music therapy governance and administration in New Zealand (1974 to 2016). *New Zealand Journal of Music Therapy 14*:10-24.

Forster, E. M. (2000). *Howards End.* First published in Great Britain by Edward Warnold 1910, this edition published by Penguin Books.

Hoskyns, S. (2011). Collaborative conversations in focus group research: Music therapists reflect on combining research and practice. *New Zealand Journal of Music Therapy 9*: 32-60.

Hoskyns, S. (2014). The student practitioner-researcher as hero in her own journey – the value of a story. *Voices: A World Forum For Music Therapy, 14*(2). doi:10.15845/voices.v14i2.777

Hoskyns, S., & Roestenburg, W. (in press). Ranga wairua: Inspiration and conversation between worlds: Māori sound science healer and a Pākehā music therapist(s) share and interweave their stories (working title). In S. Hadley and A. Crooke (Eds) *Postcolonial Music Therapy.*

Jessop, M. (2014). The grand orchestra: A humanistic conceptualization of group music therapy in dementia care. *Canadian Journal of Music Therapy ∞ Revue canadienne de musicothérapie, 20*(1): 49-64.

Kenny, C. (2006). *Music and life in the field of play*. Gilsum NH: Barcelona Publishers.

Ledger, A., & Edwards, J. (2011). Arts-based research practices in music therapy research: Existing and potential developments. *The Arts in Psychotherapy 38*: 312–317.

Ledger, A., & McCaffrey, T. (2015). Performative, arts-based, or arts-informed? Reflections on the development of arts-based research in music therapy. *Journal of Music Therapy 52*(4): 441-456.

Lorde, A. (1984). Poetry is not a luxury. In *Sister outsider: Poems and speeches by Audre Lorde* (pp. 36-39). New York: The Crossing Press.

Ministry of Health, (2017). Retrieved from: http://www.health.govt.nz/our-work/populations/maori-health/maori-health-models/maori-health-models-te-wheke

Molyneux, C. (2013). *Different perspectives – a common goal: Reflections on ten years of the Raukatauri Music Therapy Centre*. New Zealand School of Music Conference 'Linking cultures: Collaborative partnerships in music therapy and related disciplines', Wellington, New Zealand, November 2013.

Molyneux, C., Talmage, A., & McGann, H. (2016). A Music Therapy New Zealand report on music therapy provision in New Zealand. *New Zealand Journal of Music Therapy 14*: 25-54.

NiaNia, W., Bush, A., & Epston, D. (2017). *Collaborative and indigenous mental health therapy: Tātaihono – Stories of Māori healing and psychiatry*. New York: Routledge.

Nicol, J. (2008). Creating vocative texts. *The Qualitative Report 13*(3): 316-333.

Pavlicevic, M. (1999). *Music therapy: Intimate notes*. London: Jessica Kingsley Publishers.

Pere, R. (1997). *Te wheke: A celebration of infinite wisdom (2nd Edition)*. Wairoa: Ao Ako Global Learning New Zealand.

Rickson, D., Castelino, A., Molyneux, C., Ridley, H., & Upjohn-Beatson, E. (2016). What evidence? Designing a mixed methods study to investigate music therapy with children who have autism spectrum disorder (ASD), in New Zealand contexts. *The Arts in Psychotherapy 50*: 119-125.

Rickson, D., Molyneux, C., Ridley, H., Castelino, A., & Upjohn-Beatson, E. (2015). Music therapy with people who have autism spectrum disorder: Current practice in New Zealand. *New Zealand Journal of Music Therapy 13*: 8-32.

Rickson, D., & Skewes McFerran, K. (2014). *Creating music cultures in the schools: A perspective from community music therapy*. Gilsum NH: Barcelona Publishers.

Rollo, T. M. P. (2013). Mā te wai ka piki ake te hauora. *New Zealand Journal of Music Therapy 11*: 51-80.

Rykov, M. H. (2007). Dear Mr. Rilke: An arts-informed contemplation. *The Arts in Psychotherapy, 34*(5): 379-387.

Rykov, M. (2011). Writing music therapy. *Voices: A World Forum For Music Therapy, 11*(1). doi:10.15845/voices.v11i1.288

Talmage, A., Ludlam, S., Leão, S., Fogg, L., & Purdy, S. (2013). Leading the CeleBRation Choir: The Choral Singing Therapy protocol and the role of the music therapist in a social singing group for adults with neurological conditions. *New Zealand Journal of Music Therapy 11*: 7-50.

Twyford, K. (2013). Introducing time defined Specialist Music Therapy Services within the Ministry of Education Special Education, NZ: Outcomes from a pilot project study. *New Zealand Journal of Music Therapy 11*: 104-132.

Warren, P., & Rickson, D. (2016). What factors shape a music therapist? An investigation of music therapists' professional identity over time in New Zealand. *New Zealand Journal of Music Therapy 14*: 55-81.

Winterson, J. (2011). *Why be happy when you could be normal?* London: Jonathan Cape.

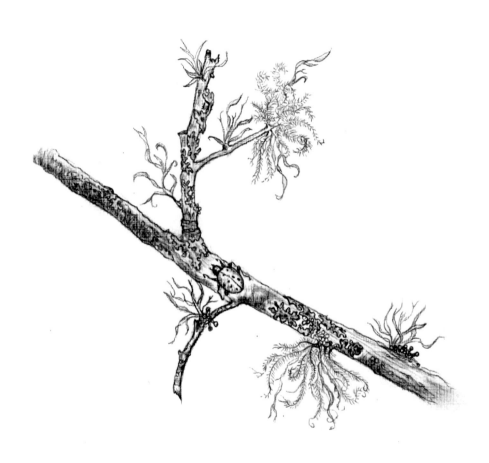

I

The Therapy Room

The door to the therapy room

Claire Molyneux

The door to the therapy room is open. In fact, all three therapy rooms are empty of people, waiting for the next clients to arrive. And yet the rooms themselves are not empty, but waiting, full of potential; unspoken interaction and connection that is yet to occur keenly anticipated or anxiously awaited.

Standing at the open door to the large therapy room, my eyes are drawn round the room by a trail of instruments. On the floor a little distance from the door is a djembe turned on its side, its large round face towards me and colourful body out behind. I wonder: will the child coming into this room go to this drum first – will they strike the skin with their hand or sit astride the drum? Next to the djembe a floor tom stands; stout and sturdy with legs set low. A beater rests on top of the tom, the handle tantalisingly close, inviting me to play. A low bench next, dark in colour and with a large mallet on top, its thick wooden handle leading to a broad felt head. Ah … this can be used to play the cymbal. I observe the cymbal; the legs of the tripod stand set wide, cymbal angled low. I can see here the therapist's care and attention: the bench positioned so the child can support himself with one hand and play with the other; the large mallet, slightly unwieldy for him, but enabling him to stretch and develop strength and coordination; the softness of the large felt head offering some tactile comfort maybe.

The piano is next. No stool for this child – he stands to play, his chin barely reaching the keys. I can imagine the therapist kneeling next to him, delighting in his independence. Will he use one or both hands to sound the keys on the piano? Further on from the piano, underneath the large windows, sits a large brightly coloured gathering drum. A smaller drum next to it and a smaller one still next to that. Windchimes, a basket of percussion, and finally the guitar brings us back to the door. The guitar, poised to play the goodbye song, marking the transition from this creative space back into the arms of a waiting parent.

The second room is small. A piano stands at the end wall, next to the window. In the centre of the room a group of standing percussion: gathering drum, floor tom, cymbal, tone blocks. A single pair of soft beaters. To one side the xylophone is waiting, silently, the blue and red castanets positioned on top of the bars. A single pair of egg shakers sit in a basket. The guitar on its stand by the window. The blind lowered just enough to stem the glare of the afternoon sun.

What will it be first? The drum? Checking to see if I remembered the egg shakers? Some negotiation outside the room to try and bring in a new instrument? And what will my role be? To play, to watch, to illuminate? Each moment brings opportunity and challenge, the instruments tools in the lively process of playful interaction between me and my client. He sees me as a distraction from the real process of mastering each instrument in a way only he knows the rules for. How can I stay close to his experience while inviting him to share mine?

Moving on, I come to the third room. A large colourful drum sits on the floor in the centre of the room. A pair of egg shakers are positioned on top of the drum. A bench to one side and the guitar leaning against the wall – no stand this time. The large drum is offered as a central space for play and gathering. I imagine the fragile and tentative dance that takes place around this drum, the attempts to create space for play and connection amongst the ever-present demand for sameness and routine.

The therapy room is so much more than a neutral space waiting to be filled. Brimming with anticipation or anxiety, I plan and hope, try to create an inviting space while holding my expectations in check. This space is sometimes my place of refuge, where I steal a few quiet moments before my client arrives, finding in myself the stillness that is needed before I can be fully present with the other.

I am reminded of an articulate young woman I worked with many years ago who was trying to integrate a traumatic experience in her life. We sat together in a room on the first floor of the purpose-built unit where I worked. I had taken care to position the instruments casually in the room, not too many expectations here. As we sat together, the unsounded instruments became louder and louder, clamouring for attention. The silence between us, punctuated by the occasional verbal exchange, felt too loud, too scary, but seemed the only thing possible. I tried to stay curious, taking my feelings of inadequacy, fear and frustration to supervision to better understand what was emerging in this silent relationship. For several weeks we sat with the instruments in this way, until one week I invited her to help me put them all away. The noise of our movements, our contact with the instruments, broke the silence and a tentative exploration of sound and surface emerged. What relief! We both realised here was something we could build on, a foundation of sound, beyond the painful silence.

Not a cupboard

Marie Willis

Not a 'cupboard' or a cluttered classroom full of distractions that therapists make-do with, but a corner room with a view is what we were given to turn into a music-place, for one day every week. It was next to the library of all places, however, we were welcomed to make whatever noise we wished, in the pursuit of connection, catharsis and collaboration.

The ritual of creating a space to receive people, their sounds and stories, began well before the nine o'clock bell; moving tables and chairs, re-setting the clock whose new battery seemed to stop week after week when the music wasn't there!

Five past nine on the dot, the 'ting' of the lift bell would announce the arrival of the first eager musicians. Just time to secure the 'please do not disturb' sign to the door before a group of young folk tumbled over the threshold. Some sang as they detoured amongst the library books and were ushered along by a friendly hand, some raced for the instrument basket, eager to peruse the plethora of objects that lay silently waiting to be struck or shaken, even stirred.

Sometimes cacophony, sometimes quiet calm; the day was filled with different musical journeys. Some preferred silence or to listen to my musicking, my song, my comments, my call to action. Some attuned to the traffic outside, the planes overhead, the calls of boys playing rugby on the field next door. Some seemed to hear the tick of the clock above any sounds I made. Sometimes that tick-tock seemed overwhelming when waiting, wondering; sometimes almost willing a person to play. Sometimes we settled for songs about the rain and the seagulls that made rhythms on our roof.

The routine of preparation and reconfiguration occurred five times daily; each 'creative customer' requiring a different assortment of instruments, spaces and considerations. Chairs would be rearranged or removed, drum kits wheeled out and xylophones wheeled in. Alcohol wipes were recruited for cleaning a whole manner of things, and new beaters sought to replace those that flew out of the window.

The music did not remain in 'the music room'. Oh no, it travelled along corridors; woven on journeys to reach, and return from that musicking place. Connections often began outside the door; on the playground swings or in the tuneful 'hello' of the staff in the hall. Music was shared by all folk in this place and brought smiles and delight to many a face. And years since I've gone, some have moved on, and yet the music still lives there and plays on and on.

I walk into the room

Carolyn Ayson

I walk into the room. I see the spot by the TV where I will place the guitar for the child to unpack. In the corner waits a pile of instruments, untouched since this time last week. The TV, in my absence, provided music with programmes like 'The Voice' for her to sing along to. A wooden chair has been carefully placed beside the couch in anticipation of me coming. The child knows that this is her place to sit. Its four legs centre and ground her. She will warm it for 40 minutes. This family room is always changing. Coffee cups come and go. Our music will take place beside the folded washing: connecting with everyday life, becoming part of it.

A golden-hued piano

Nolan Hodgson

A golden-hued piano dominates the music room. Its scuffed and graffitied surface belies a well-prepared interior. The strings are tuned and hammers ready to flood the room with a rich sound that can hold its own against the drum kit opposite. There is also a pair of guitars who live here intermittently. Popular with staff and patients alike, these guitars often wander down hallways and are found in people's rooms. They're commonly seen swapping songs in shared lounges and are sometimes secreted away in offices down the hall. The drum kit appears a bit three-legged at first, waiting patiently in the corner with a few saggy skins and a weary crash cymbal. In spite of this, the adolescents who frequent this room know how to warm into it and can conjure up a turbulent fury of rhythm if they fancy. The kit welcomes these encounters, accepting them as readily as it does a few timid strokes from someone who has never held a drumstick in their life.

The room itself is slight with pale walls. A double window overlooks an internal courtyard with a shaggy vege garden. The door is locked whenever the room is empty and it has a window in the top half so people can see inside without interrupting. Lining a box in the corner and spread atop the piano are an erratic array of music scores and handwritten compositions. Books of nursery rhymes, scores from musicals and other well known pieces intermingle with original songs and poems scrawled into notebooks. These are the viscera of thoughts and emotions that people propel into living, breathing moments of sound in this room.

While the music room itself is small, it is animated by the presence and history of the instruments. The piano has accompanied rap, honed classical repertoire and bashed out pop melodies for choruses of young singers. Teenagers have refined beats on the drum kit and churned out messy rhythms in time with their favourite tunes. The guitars have been composed on and collaborated with by pairs of new friends and wary acquaintances. Together the instruments have played in hundreds of ensembles, impromptu jams and evening talent-quest mash-ups.

For people staying in this unit of the hospital, this room is at their disposal. They can choose to practise in it quietly or announce themselves dramatically. Either way, they allow their music to drift out through the open door and share the vitality it carries with anyone within earshot. As a music therapist, it is a joy to share in these experiences and a challenge to tailor and encourage musical interactions that benefit the health of everyone involved. While the music can repel people as often as it attracts them, the fact that it can reach through the wall and gain people's attention is an enormous advantage. In this sense the 'music room' is able to expand and include half the unit and multiple rooms, or even to travel in someone's hands with the guitar. Of course the little room looks bare and slightly dilapidated when empty, but this is because it has been worn-in so thoroughly. It still has plenty of life left before it will become worn-out.

Up the steep stairs
Heather Fletcher

Up the steep stairs, sandwiched between the resource room and the staff toilet is a smallish rectangular room called the 'Play Room'. But there's not much to play with in here. The room is empty except for some wall-mounted cupboards and a floor-standing cupboard, bolted to the wall. The room is full of light, which is streaming in through the windows that fill the long wall. Luckily there are blinds to shade the light when it becomes too intense … although some of these are broken. There are metal grills covering the heater, intended to keep careless or inquisitive hands safe from being burned. However, the grill becomes just as hot when the heater is on. There is well-worn carpet on the floor and the walls are bare. This is the blank canvas from which the therapist must conjure a safe and interesting space in which to welcome the client.

I need to think ahead. In winter, I warm the room up before parents arrive with their child, then turn the heaters off so they are cooling down during the session. Safer for little hands. I place a brightly coloured giant cushion in front of the heater. In the summer, I open all the windows ahead of the session … to cool the room down. I close them again before we start, to prevent the smaller instruments ending up in the car park below.

There is a reason the room is bare. It is used by a variety of clinicians, each needing different equipment for their work. If we all filled it with our toys, instruments or furniture, the room would be cluttered and distracting. It used to be like this but now each of us just brings in what we need ... and takes it away again when we've finished. This way we can focus on what's important.

So, what do I need? Today, it needs to be simple and robust. Smaller instruments and beaters are out - they too easily get lobbed around the room or used to hit the walls. I do need drums though, so I bring in three: two tabla and a bodhran. Next some windchimes on a stand. And finally my guitar. That's not much, but I haven't finished yet. A bright pink Swiss ball, a large multi-coloured scarf and some soft toy animals.

Now I am ready. Let the fun begin.

The room is warm
Shari Storie

The room is warm, a muted smell of the day before. Reluctantly, because it means the natural light cannot come in, I have kept the windows and blinds closed; to minimise noise and visual distraction from the car park just outside, to minimise the visual distraction of bands of shadows on the walls and floor or the breeze blowing the blinds, and to provide some privacy for those inside the room. And so the small room is filled with artificial white light on creamy-yellow walls covered with brightly coloured posters and artwork. Not the most ideal but the most appropriate room available, this space holds the people and the music that has come before, and is ready for more to come.

At 9:30 am I begin to ready the room. Table moved to one end, chairs to the other, stray nails collected off the floor, sensory toys and beanbag cleared into the sensory room next door. Instruments in from the car. More chairs sought from other rooms. By 10:10 am I stand at the door, surveying the room, checking everything is in place, running through my session plan in my mind. I have kept the two chairs in the middle of the room, with a guitar between facing the door; the first and most consistent place we'll travel to once inside the room. I have stretched the lycra over a few select instruments on the far table, to assess my client's attention span with minimal visual distraction. The few instruments selected don't have any strings or cords and are ready to test palmar grasp, pincer grip and fine motor skills. The xylophone table, the tall conga drum, the cymbal and floor tom are placed in different corners of the room to enable travel, distance, proximity and standing play.

10:55 am and the wooden table at one end of the room now has an array of instruments laid out in categories. Different coloured tambourines in a line on one side, various shakers in a line along the front with the handles sticking out just over the edge inviting and awaiting selection. Assorted drums sit in one corner next to the table, and in the corner opposite are tuned percussion on odd tables and side-turned drawers. A circle of chairs is ready near the door at the other end of the room. The keyboard is on its stand nestled along one wall, just far enough away from the reach of those about to sit on the chairs.

12:30 pm. I have opened the windows to cool the room, as this next client won't stay if the room is too warm. Fewer instruments this time, the engaging focal points being the windchimes at one end, the keyboard along the side, the xylophone opposite and a few small percussion on the table at the other end. A ukulele, no guitar, and the keyboard tone pre-tuned to 'music box'.

1:20 pm and a quick transformation. Two rows of instruments, mostly tilted inward at an angle conducive for reaching and playing, line the centre of the room with a gap just wide enough for a wheelchair to navigate between. My flute, assembled, catches the light and I smile, anticipating the dancing and the moving, the vocalising and the drumming.

2:05 pm. Another transformation sees flute, thumb pianos and twizzle drum put away safely, and out come the sturdy bongos. Aligned back to back on the bright red table, chairs opposite, ready for shared yet independent play. The keyboard by the door, ready to welcome and greet through song, the guitar opposite, awaits farewell .

2:50 pm and I scramble to clean everything with medi-wipes one final time. Instruments back into their cases and out to the car. Ideally by 3:00 pm, but often not until 3:10 pm, I stand at the door double-checking I have everything, pressing on to my next port of call.

The space breathes and holds the diverse people and music of the day, and will be ready again next week.

At first glance

Libby Johns

At first glance the child and I see four walls covered with educational posters and children's art. We smell a slightly stale aroma from a lack of ventilation throughout the day. The fluorescent tube lights flicker on and we awaken the old classroom. The large windows on two opposing walls stare at one another, their old venetian blinds have long tatty cords that look as though they have been pulled hard one too many times. There is old carpet, thin and navy blue, stained after years of service. The wall heater is small and loud as it takes fifteen minutes to warm the room. The whiteboard covers fifty percent of one wall and lists the days of the week in te reo, types of weather, and several smudged names of students who have been singled out for an unknown reason. Old instruments are placed off to the side, the large ones covered in cloth and the others out of sight in the attached office. We spread our instruments out keeping a walking path between the wall and our instruments of choice. Last week we created an imaginary boundary within the room using only a small portion of floor space, today we are spread far and wide. This well-loved space is ready for another adventure; always welcoming the sounds and interaction we offer, incredibly resilient to that which we ask of it. Withholding judgement through all the action, emotion and challenge in our session, it never whispers a word.

At the end of the day

Alison Talmage

Here I am after the last goodbye song, as the day's rhythm slows. After the cycle of hello songs, improvisations, farewells, note writing, readying for the next greeting, session, connection. Each instrument sings me its memories, plays with my emotions, suggests a next time. Drums stand silent now, but I still hear exuberant, playful beats. A xylophone, bars askew, conjures up fragments of melody. Small percussion instruments spill out of a basket next to hollows in the pillows where we sat to shake, click, tap the maracas, castanets, tambourine. I gather carefully lined up drumsticks and retrieve others discarded by a shorter attention span. Wipe away fingermarks from favourite instruments, wondering whether they'll share next time, play something else one day. Let the windchimes resound, evoking a child's stretch, smile, shared delight. Retune the guitar. Strum, hum, jot down lyrics and chords while I remember. Transcribe improvisation fragments, motifs we might explore again. On the piano I doodle possibilities, then close the lid, close the door. I file my notes, but the children's songs remain in my mind and mine in theirs.

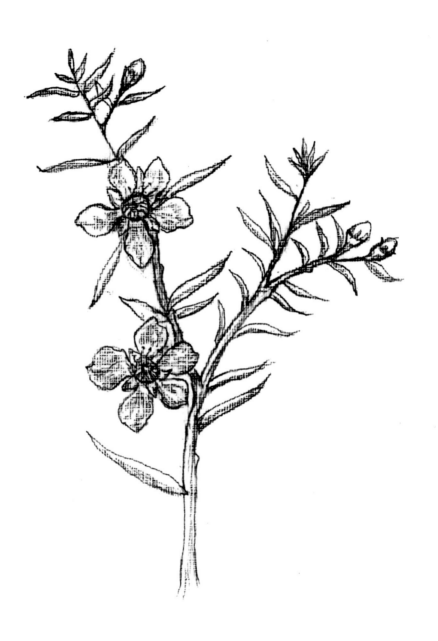

II
Poems and Stories
from Music Therapy

Let the Children Teach You

Alison Talmage

'Let the children teach you' – the words of music therapy pioneer Clive Robbins, during his final visit to Auckland in 2007. Through spontaneous play – musical, physical, imaginative, solitary, collaborative - children reveal their joys, strengths and difficulties. Children's worlds are not neatly divided by subject boundaries. Many children arrive at the music therapy room with an expectation that singing, playing and dancing will be at the heart of our work together. Others find a wonderful space for running, climbing, hiding, pretend play, or a place that they don't initially understand and would prefer to exit. I meet children with extensive experience of music, others with none. Children with extensive song repertoires, others just beginning to explore their voices. Children who can create and sustain complex rhythm patterns, others with a barely emerging sense of pulse. Children who sound the xylophone bars in order, up and down, down and up; others who take the instrument apart and line up bars and beaters on the floor. I love to see children's play through children's eyes, to enter their world as well as inviting them into a world of music, to extend their capacity for play, self-expression, self-regulation and relationships.

When child-centredness comes first, music-centred play may be immediate or may gradually emerge. Inviting children to participate, rather than directing, gives them permission to bring themselves more fully into the music therapy room. Framing my role as witness and play partner, or listener and fellow musician, means emphasising safety, music, relationships, but also following the children's interests.

This collection of poems recalls experiences of music therapy with children with autism, who have difficulty connecting with other people and the world around them. All the children depicted are composite characters, to protect individual identities. The poems illustrate my understanding that all behaviour is communication, and portray children as active players, however tentative or dynamic, from the start of our work together.

Beginning 1

alert	curious
self-absorbed	I sing your name
eyes averted	watch
muscles tense	softly
circling, tiptoeing	mark your footsteps
hugging the walls	reach tentatively into
keeping your distance	the space between
wailing suddenly	I breathe in … out …
you rush close	surprised
slam the piano shut	hear your fear
snatch my drumsticks	give you space
push the xylophone	keep you safe
cover your ears	listen
retreat	wait
into echoing silence	before singing again
avoiding contact	inviting hope
some people	I
concerned, anxious	patiently
might take your hand	show you how my hands
and sit you down	tap rhythms
and make you play	sound melodies
and tell you how to be	suggest possibilities
hurry you to do the same	take time to understand
be the same	your uniqueness
as everyone	your voice
slowly	gradually
this space	here
will seem safer	trust will grow
with eyes and ears open	we will both learn
you will edge closer to me	to play together
the piano, drum, xylophone	new sounds, colours, thoughts

sounding our selves
making new songs
connecting
becoming

Beginning 2

A child-sized whirlwind hurtles through the door spins twizzles twirls turns discards shoes socks jersey *we keep our shirts on in the music room* bag books toys except for the one indispensable thing that can't possibly wait in Mum's bag for later so we'll drive it into the music room *let's go, the wheels on the bus go round and round, round and round, round and round …* round the room whizzing whirling *here we are in the music room* squeezing behind the piano *you and me in the music room* reappearing hurrying scurrying bounding *pounding drumbeats matching footsteps* won't stop can't stop *after sitting sitting sitting in class in the car in the rush hour* rush past fast cast a glance *good to see you today* left right left right *drum cymbal crash splash* running jumping leaping *in time with you* laughing loving the fun the freedom the feeling of being alive *slowing down as you drift to the corner* dragging the chair across the room *moving closer keeping you safe* clambering up gazing out of the window *we are inside looking outside* jump down up again *inside looking outside* down round and round *we are dancing* round and round *the driver on the bus says please sit down* crouching *sit down here* crawling *here we are in the music room* sitting *here we are together.*

The big gathering drum is …

my voice
calling, yelling,
telling you I'm here

a hiding place
when I feel playful,
cheerful, sorrowful

a wheel
driving across the room
from you to me

a sailing boat
braving stormy seas
while you sing me safely home

a gymnast's springboard
when I climb, count, jump,
and you catch me

anything I imagine
somewhere we share music
and more.

Improvisation

One
sound, then
twos and threes,
my melody steps, leaps, repeats.
I see motifs, play phrases,
clusters in the spaces,
I find sounds and silence,
clashing discords and gentle harmony.
Listen, listen, listen
before you sing me your song.

I love watching and listening to spontaneous piano playing by young children, including those who have autism. Children are curious about the orderly layout of the keyboard with its intriguing asymmetry of black keys in pairs and threes, and the predictable left to right, low to high sounds. I have listened to endless scales, up and down, up and down on every white key, then up and down, up and down on every black key. While I might worry about rigid thinking and the child's reluctance to let me join in, I believe this free exploration also signifies a sense of control, self-confidence and creativity.

While improvisational music therapy encourages exploration and free play, with no need for theoretical knowledge, some readers who are not pianists might like to refer to the keyboard diagram that shows the repeated A-G labelling of the white keys and dual naming of the black keys as higher ('sharp' or #) and lower ('flat' or ♭) than the adjacent keys.

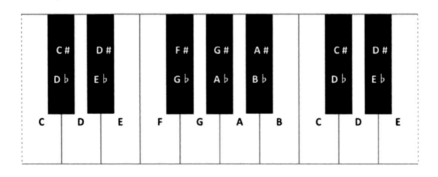

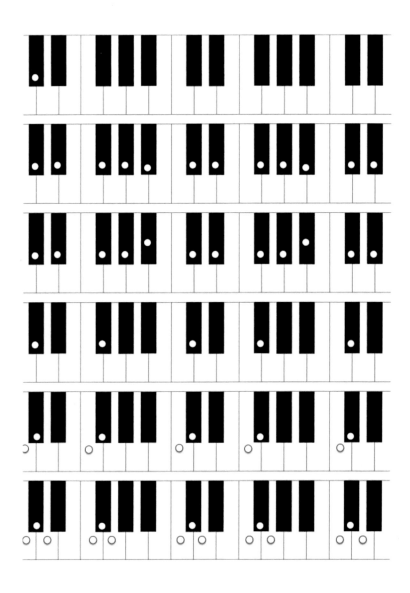

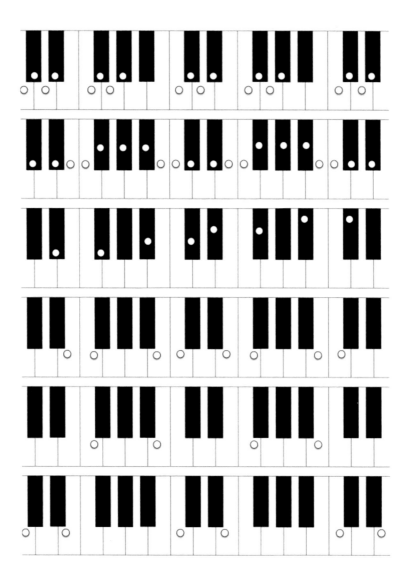

Things I like in the music room

Round things for tapping, banging, hitting,
And a shiny circle for crashing, splashing, spinning.

The huge round sound of a sea storm,
And the small round jingly not-quite-a-drum.

Twelve wooden squarish sticks lined up on a box,
And more long, short, thick, thin sticks for lining up on the floor or
        making noise.

Long strings on funny shaped boxes
To pull, twang, stroke, strum.

Red orange yellow green blue turquoise purple white red again
things to shake and ring,
Red orange yellow green blue turquoise purple white red again
boxes sounding the same.

The giant thing with a hiding place behind,
In front the black and white noise-makers.

The person who plays and lets me play,
Sings, shares, shows and lets me try,
And knows the names of these favourite things.

The Notebook

Claire Molyneux

Five years old. Normal birth and delivery. Quiet, placid baby. Preschool teacher first to raise concern; autism, developmental delay. First-born. No siblings to make a comparison. At 18 months, no language, did not respond to name. Little eye contact. Very active, climbing, no sense of danger. Loves music. Always responds to familiar songs. As a baby would rock and bounce in time. Gets upset when music is played or when parents sing particular songs. Attends preschool. Doesn't play with other children.

'My boy', she told me, 'has no words.' But his communication ran much deeper than words. His gaze, albeit infrequent, was filled with intent.

'My boy', she told me, 'plays alone at kindy, he doesn't mix with the other children … but he watches them.'

The boy lies on the floor of the therapy room. His back is against the wall in a space he has chosen that is just big enough for his body but not his legs which stretch out into the room. Above him there is a window and where he lies is a heating vent. Fascinated by the vent, he closes his eyes to feel the warm air on his face and hair. His mother sits close, but not too close. He would have to move to touch her. I watch him for several minutes, waiting to see if he is interested in my presence. The space and time feel quietly peaceful, without expectation, just trying out different ways of being in each other's presence. The boy's mother is accepting of this and watches too, smiling at me occasionally. I move a drum closer and tap tentatively, testing the sound created in the space between us. The sound is quiet but enough to break his reverie and I wonder if I have interrupted too soon. He looks at me briefly before returning to focus on the warm air. I sound the drum again with my fingertips, a trickle of taps, then pause and wait … another trickle, pause and wait. The boy moves his hand on the carpet. I feel a spark of excitement and remind myself to hold the space and quiet that exists between us. I move my hand on the drum, pause and wait. He moves his fingers on the carpet and darts a look at me with his dark eyes. An invitation? I move my hand over the drum skin again and he does the same on the floor. I tap the drum and as I lift my fingers off, I hold my hand palm up, waiting. The boy taps the floor with his fingertips – a definite movement this time followed by another glance at me. I slowly ease myself into the space we have created, moving a little closer and sustaining the fragile connection that is emerging.

'My boy', she told me, 'doesn't show interest in other people, he doesn't respond to his name.'

The sounds we create, mine resonant and full on the drum, his muffled on the carpet, grow to fill the space. His posture shifts as he lifts himself up on one elbow to get a better look at me and the drum. Over the next seven minutes, the boy moves closer to me, touches the drum, holds my gaze.

'He's never done that with someone he's just met', she said. 'Usually he just ignores other people and carries on with his own thing.'

She tells me of the strategies they have put in place at preschool to support his play with others. She tells me of the routine they follow at home to help him learn basic tasks, the way she urges him to find ways to connect within the rote learning that he is capable. This boy can put puzzle pieces in the correct places, he can sort shapes, he has clear musical preferences. Yet his autism prevents him from engaging in these activities with others.

In the session, I tell him that we've finished with the drum and that I'm going to get the guitar. My chest tightens as I reach for the guitar; is the connection we created with the drum strong enough to sustain a change like this? The boy moves back a fraction, pressing his body against the wall. I wonder if my movements are too fast and I remind myself to breathe and move slowly. I nestle the guitar on my lap. I glance at the boy, then at the guitar. I don't notice my eyebrows rising until his do too.

With my fingertips, I tap the body of the guitar, round the edge, brushing over the strings, making them vibrate inaudibly. I watch my hand as it moves. Stopping, I hold it palm out and glance at the boy, barely lifting my head. He moves his hand on the carpet. Off I go again, tapping the guitar body, teasing out rhythms, increasing in speed and intensity, then stop. This time, the boy moves his hand before I even have a chance to look up. Closer this time, sending my fingers dancing on the guitar, brushing across the strings as I gain confidence that these new sounds are going to be okay in the space between us. My chest relaxes and I feel a smile. This time his hand is there just before I stop playing, hovering in the air between us. He pushes my hand back and I feel a rush of excitement as my fingers touch the strings and away I go again, playing louder this time. The physical contact between us grows stronger and surer with each pause and return, the boy pushing my hand back to the strings to sustain the music. I am suddenly aware of his mother, watching lovingly, smiling as her boy communicates his intentions, his hand dancing in the musical space we have created. On the next turn, I pause longer and hold my hand out. As he puts his fingers in mine, I bring his hand to the strings. Too much? I glance at his mother. Her eyes fill with tears. A moment of unexpected communication, unexpected connection. Suddenly overwhelmed the boy looks to his mother for comfort. She offers her lap and from here he is able to hold my gaze, touching my hand when I pause, returning it to the guitar in an effort to sustain the music. He puts his hand in mine again and allows me to bring his fingers to the guitar, his touch strong enough to sound the strings this time. He leaves his hand there.

Relaxed he glances at Mum and back to the guitar. It is time for us to finish. He has given as much as he can for today, invited me in just far enough. The three of us rest in the knowledge that this rare connection heralds more possibilities. There is hope as he sits back on Mum's lap, his body folding in on itself, tired from the exertion of simply being with, but watching as I replace the guitar and fetch my notebook from the top of the piano.

A Relationship Remembered Through Fragments

Claire Molyneux

Jesse has this funny habit of pushing his lips out as if he is trying to make his top lip touch his nose. When he does this, he looks at me … I wonder what he is sensing or responding to. I try it and feel the way it stretches my top lip – is this a way of releasing tension? It feels like a question mark to me in a funny sort of way as it makes my eyes wrinkle up too. What might the question be? For me, it seems to be one of how to connect, how to share a space together, how to come to a place of understanding. I wonder what the question is for Jesse.

Here are some of the things I remember about Jesse in music therapy:

You wanting to get as close as possible to me, holding my hands to make me sound the instruments.

Your desire for skin to skin contact. You would press your arm into the space between my chin and neck or take my arm and put it under your chin. On Friday mornings when I dressed, I would do so with an awareness of my session with you, wearing a shirt with a collar, knowing that certain items of clothing elicited more body contact from you than others. Why was this important? Because as a pre-adolescent, it was important for you to learn boundaries to keep yourself and others safe.

Your jumping. Not necessarily to the music, but to an internal drive. I could use this movement to inform the music I played; directing dynamics, attack, duration. I wondered if it was a relief when the internal drive to jump was transformed into the action of striking the cymbal or drum. The instrument giving voice to the energy inside of you and generating a way we could dialogue and share that energy. I saw sometimes that this lessened your need to jump as you became more interested in our playing or the landing of the beater as it struck the drum skin.

Your response to piano music. Sometimes I felt that the music I produced on the piano and with my voice was not big enough to hold whatever it was that needed to be expressed. Full harmonies, sweeping melodies, a sense of urgency to find the power that could hold the intensity of feeling and expression that I sensed. And it was a sensing, something that I cannot explain objectively, but became subject to in the relationship with you. Was I a conduit? Expressing the music within you through some dynamic transference? Playing what you could not play, the music giving voice to all that you wanted to say? And how much was my own music present? The music surely contained something for us both in that moment; for me a willing for the music to be big enough and full enough to hold an unspoken need, expressed through my fingers, every synapse in my brain engaged in embodying and expressing what I was aware of in the room. I remember feeling that my voice could never be powerful enough to express the emotion present. And yet, there was a fine balance between this vibrant, full and passionate expression and you being tipped into a place of overwhelm, the sensory input too much.

Actually, it was these moments that intrigued me. Some sessions could be full of powerful, loud expression to which you responded with smiles and playing and returning my hands to the piano to continue. At other times, your response was more edgy, you bit your hand or grabbed my arm, squeezing it hard. We called this dysregulation, but I suspect it was your way of trying to let me know something. In those moments I fell woefully short of understanding; did we need to move into the dysregulation to better understand and explore it together or did we need to find a more centred space? I think each time the need may have been different. There were times when you seemed to want me to just play, the same guitar chord progression over and over, adding my voice. If I stopped, you would return my hand to the strings. This seemed to be calming for you, creating a meditative space, one where we were able to share the experience of being present in the room, listening to the music, sitting close side by side.

I remember turn-taking exchanges. Sharing the lollipop drums, we took turns to hold them for each other to play. You wanted to bang them together and I showed you how to hold them for me to play. I had to play them hard to create the resonance that satisfied you. While I was aware of the extrinsic pull of the goal here (turn-taking and sharing with others), there was so much playfulness between us – let me try and describe it:

You walked over to the table and picked up the two drums shaped like lollipops with a colourful swirly pattern on the drum part and a red handle, one smaller than the other. Holding one in each hand, you hit them together, hard, creating a boomy, resonant sound. Your eyes found mine and I saw your smile.

Internally, I felt my concern for the instruments. Could the drums stand up to being bashed together like this, was there a different way we could create the same sound? But even more importantly, how could I join in with you? Your smile seemed to be an invitation and you accepted me standing next to you. I held my hand out for one of the drums and you passed it to me. I gave you one of the brightly coloured beaters and took the other one myself. I played the drum with the beater and touched your hand to encourage you to do the same. No, this wasn't going to work, too much direction, not enough playfulness. I held my hand out for the other beater and gave you both drums. Again you bashed them together, smiled and looked at me, that delightful invitation again: 'Go on then!' I showed you how to hold them out for me to play. It is so difficult to convey in words, the exchange that occurred here. You knew my intention, you understood your role in this game we were creating together: you held the drums and I played. Then I held the drums and you played. But that simple exchange does not convey the delight communicated in the action. We both hit the drums hard, so hard that occasionally one or other of us would lose our grip and we'd have to pick them up off the floor. The different sized drums produced different pitches. A two-tone melody was created, a shared pulse sustained. This play was so much more than taking turns. We were engaged in play that generated musical sound and structure, facilitated shared joy and pleasure. Both of us participated with commitment and energy until the exchange fell apart and the drums were returned to the table.

Your thunder-claps. The percussive sound *thwack!* as you clapped your hands together in front of your open mouth. I couldn't quite imitate it, and can't find quite the right word to represent the sound on paper. I would experiment with my hands and my mouth: if I open it like this, place my hands just here, palms touching or a small space between where my hands come together with a swift movement. You watched, anticipating my failure. Then you would demonstrate again and I was lost for response, save a look in my eyes that said 'Show me again.' And you would:

> I offered my hands in response and you raised your hands to mine. *Clap!* You held my gaze, a forthright invitation to eye contact. Your eyes smiled and I offered my hands again. We stood face to face, hand to hand. Hands moved out and back, to and fro, just enough repetition to see if the rhythm had a momentum of its own. I made bigger movements with my arms, sustaining the pulse we were seeking, extending each moment of anticipation and satisfying resolve as your hands hit mine.
>
> You shrieked, all the while holding my gaze in this game of pat-a-cake. I responded with my voice; not quite a shriek, but trying to match the intensity of your vocalisation. Our movements quickened, becoming smaller. You came closer and I held for a moment then took a big step away, hoping you might follow, aiming to add movement to our intense exchange, aiming to sustain the moment before it became overwhelming and the pulse collapsed.

I remember the drums. We played the djembe together. Taking turns, you would play first, tapping with your fingers, sometimes using the back of your fingers, flicking one against the other. I responded, trying to find a rhythm, a pulse. You understood this turn-taking, you could wait and respond, listen to me play then have your turn.

Your play with beaters. At first these were objects to pick up and drop, later they became objects to put in my hand, taking my arm to make me sound the drum or cymbal. I encouraged you to hold the beater and you did, sometimes with help, sometimes independently. I remember the long periods of improvisation we had when you played the drum and cymbal and I played the piano. You wanted to hold the beaters in just one hand and I would prompt you to 'Use both hands'. You did. The music would gradually find a sustained pulse, grow in intensity and then would pause, faltering until we started again. There was joy when we found ways to play together without these interruptions.

I remember when you first waved the beaters in my face. I flinched, a reflex, then my conscious mind interpreted the event and I decided there was no danger in your action, you merely wanted to see my face behind the flickering movement of the beaters. Sometimes you became mischievous, turning from the drum to use the beaters on the piano keys, looking at me as you did so, knowing that this was something I would re-direct. I celebrated your mischief, but was bound by the need to model appropriate behaviour. I didn't mind how you used the beaters, but not on the piano keys which were liable to chip when bashed!

I remember your emotional connection with the music. The way a sudden moment of tears within a piano improvisation, a shriek or laugh, could come out of nowhere. It felt as if the music contained you, literally you were in the music, the music gave voice and sound to your feelings, to our feelings in the moment.

I remember our goodbye song with the guitar. It felt important to sit together at the end of the session and yet I know this was hard for you in the beginning. When you noticed I had learned a new chord progression, one that you really liked, we were able to create a song from this. A song that we used many times: times when you cried while I played; times when you played yourself, strumming the strings and sometimes hitting them with the palm of your hand; and times when you returned my hand to the strings, showing some frustration as you implored me to just keep playing rather than invite you to play. You wanted to listen. Other times, you put the guitar away, almost as soon as we started to play, or pushed it out of my hands.

These are the things I remember about our work together. I could, and have presented this work as a case study at a conference. I could write it up for publication, use an acceptable format, making sure I cover all the essential details such as your age, diagnosis, reason for referral, goals and outcomes of the therapeutic intervention. Or I could offer a remembering of our work through prose that tries to capture the energy, commitment and intensity of the musical relationship, that honours the human connection and the poetic moments we shared. Prose that remembers you: Jesse, the boy to whose question I cannot put words.

Remember the Little Things
Heather Fletcher

St David of Wales, 6th Century, was a tough old wizard, much loved and respected by his flock. His dying message was 'Remember the little things that you have seen me do.'

Esylit Harker, 2008.

I have set out the room with just a few instruments; two small drums, windchimes on a stand and guitar. Potential projectiles are absent as in the past a number of the smaller instruments have ended up out the window! I have also cleared the room of tables and chairs and anything else that's interesting to climb on, so we all sit on the floor. I have learned to keep things simple. This way, we can focus on relationships. As I wait for Sammy[1] and his mum to arrive, I take a moment to reflect on our journey together and think about how I need to be with them today. I feel I need to be calm, keep verbal communication to a minimum and, above all, I need to be attentive.

I am brought into the present by a squeal from downstairs. Sammy and his mum have arrived. Sammy is keen to climb the stairs to where the sessions take place, he knows where he's going. However, today I intercept them at the foot of the stairs. We have some important business to attend to. I encourage him to sit on his bottom and shuffle up and down the first few steps. I have adapted the song *Here we go round the mulberry bush,* which I now sing, and encourage Mum to sing also: *This is the way we climb the stairs.* After practising this a few times, we allow Sammy to turn around and climb all the way up to the top, the way he usually does. He doesn't have a problem going up the stairs. I am, in fact, preparing him for the end of the session, when he needs to go down the stairs, which, up until now, has always been very traumatic for Sammy. I have no idea whether this will work, but Mum and I have agreed to give it a go. We will have to wait until the end of the session to see whether it does in fact make a difference.

Once in the therapy room, Sammy initiates our start/stop game, which he leads playing the chimes. I play a simple three-chord riff on the guitar and Mum plays the drums. We play together and Mum and I stop playing when Sammy does. He gives me a fleeting sideways glance. I take this as acknowledgement that he understands what we are doing: we are listening to him and joining him in his world. He starts to play again, swaying in time to the music. He grabs the chimes again to stop the sound; this time glancing at both of us as he does so, as if challenging us to stop playing, which we do. He lets out a small laugh and starts to play again. He begins to vary the length of time he plays before stopping. I feel like he's testing us and checking to see if he really is in control of the music. He is certainly challenging us to be attentive and responsive. Mum is finding this difficult, however, and after a few minutes she forgets to stop playing. Sammy responds by going over to Mum and rolling the drum away. It's as if he's saying: 'You're not playing by the rules, so you can't play anymore.'

I return the drum to Mum and gently remind her to stop playing when Sammy stops. We continue this game and whenever we stop playing, I gasp and look surprised. Sammy then does something quite unexpected. He comes over to me and feels my face, before returning to the game. The next time we stop playing, he copies my facial expression. It's as though just looking at me is not enough for him to understand what I am doing, but in feeling it, he is making sense of it and is able to imitate me, just as I am doing by starting and stopping with him.

My sense is that Sammy is waking up. By this, I mean that he is discovering a new way to interact with the world, and is finding this can be fun. He is becoming more curious, a key component in stimulating the desire to learn. I am thrilled by this development and feel excited.

It has taken a while to get to this point. When Sammy first started attending music therapy sessions with his mum, he would run around the room, banging on the walls, cupboards, door and wall heaters; he would climb on anything he could … and jump off, and he totally ignored both myself and Mum. The exception to this was when he wanted something. He would take Mum (usually) by the hand and pull her to the object of his attention and cry and whimper until she responded by lifting him up onto the cupboard or opened the door. Sammy has not yet developed verbal communication, although he loves to vocalise.

Very early in our work together, I realised it was important I did not allow myself to be drawn into Sammy and his mum's world, but instead modelled a different way of interacting. I reflected on the concept of Bowlby's 'secure base' (1988) and thought about how I could provide this. In the end I did something very simple: I stayed in one place, sitting on the floor while this whirlwind travelled around the room. From here, whatever sounds Sammy made I would reflect back to him, be it the number of bangs on the wall or a vocal sound; letting him know I had heard him. I would offer snippets of familiar songs, pause and wait. Over time, Sammy began to take notice of me. Sometimes he stopped what he was doing and glanced at me briefly, other times he repeated the musical phrase of the song I had sung, approximating the words. He was starting to interact with me.

Returning to our game, although I feel this is great progress, I am also somewhat uncomfortable. Sammy is focusing most of his attention on me rather than Mum, and my goal is to empower Mum and improve the relationship and interactions between her and Sammy. I need to shift the focus away from my interactions with Sammy, however much Sammy and I are enjoying them, and towards the interactions between Mum and Sammy.

Now that Mum has seen how Sammy is beginning to engage with me, I encourage her to join me in what I am doing. I invite her to stay in one place, instead of running around after Sammy all the time. This alone takes a lot of trust on her part, as one of her main concerns is Sammy's safety. Sammy appears to have no concept of danger and can be impulsive in his approach to climbing on things or experimenting with hitting and throwing things. This is why I had removed virtually everything from the room and even gone to the extent of having some wall-mounted shelves removed and a large cupboard moved away from the window. In a previous session, Sammy had used the skirting board and window ledge to climb up onto the top of this cupboard and jump off. We both had to keep our wits about us to ensure Sammy did not hurt himself. I wanted to remove these temptations and make it easier for Sammy to focus on interacting with us, as well as alleviate Mum's very real concerns around his safety.

With the safety issues addressed, we can begin to focus on the therapeutic goals. I encourage Mum to wait until Sammy approaches her before interacting with him and to only respond with as much as Sammy gives her. For example, when Sammy sings the first phrase of a song, sing only that phrase back to him. This simple change in their interactions changes the whole dynamic between them. Sammy starts going to Mum more often and initiating an activity or song. Providing Mum follows Sammy's lead and only gives back as much as he offers, Sammy continues to engage. I see the delight in her face. She is experiencing Sammy in a different way, which is so much more rewarding for both of them. I allow myself to share their delight. However, Mum can only sustain this for a little while before her enthusiasm gets the better of her and she sings the rest of the song. At this, Sammy turns away and is no longer interested in the activity. He is sending a very clear message. 'That's too much. You're overloading me and I can't cope.' I gently remind Mum to only sing what Sammy sings. He soon re-engages. After the discovery of a new skill, comes the need for repetition in order to master it. I encourage Mum to continue engaging Sammy in this game for as long as he wants to sustain it. I am pleased to notice my status shifting from being the primary focus of attention, to being a witness to Sammy and Mum's joint attention.

We segue into our peek-a-boo game, which uses the tune *Frère Jacques* with adapted lyrics commonly used by New Zealand music therapists, so it becomes:

Sammy is hiding; Sammy is hiding
Where is he? Where is he?
Sammy is hiding; Sammy is hiding
There he is!
(at which point Sammy reveals himself from under the cloth).

Mum clearly enjoys this game too, but again her enthusiasm gets the better of her and she starts to poke and tickle Sammy through the cloth as soon as we start singing the song, causing him to throw off the cloth before the end of the song. He is, however, clearly enjoying this attention, rolling around and giggling, so I sit back and observe until he has had enough and stops the game. When Sammy initiates the game again, I invite Mum to delay the poking and tickling until the last line of the song. We are richly rewarded when Sammy lies still under the cloth until the last line; at which point he pulls the cloth off to reveal himself. Not only is he now engaging in joint attention, he is also learning to sequence: lying still then revealing himself at the appropriate moment in the song. I catch myself thinking about how we can extend this game. We could take turns hiding under the cloth, hide different objects, tap the beat to the song … but these will have to wait, as we are coming to the end of the session.

After we have sung goodbye, I accompany Sammy and Mum to the top of the stairs. Usually, when we get here, Sammy refuses to go down. Even when Mum picks him up to carry him, he starts to scream and cry, turning his head away from the stairs. Initially, we thought Sammy was protesting at having to leave the session. However, his distress appeared to be triggered by the stairs rather than leaving the room. It later dawned on me that perhaps Sammy was scared to go down the stairs and I wondered whether there was an issue with his depth perception. Standing at the top of the stairs, looking down, it is a long way and does indeed look quite scary. Today, I encourage Mum not to pick up Sammy, as she usually does, but to help him sit on his bottom and shuffle down the stairs, as we had practised at the start of the session. It is an unusual sight, two adults and a toddler shuffling down the stairs on their bottoms, singing a song. But it works! Sammy successfully gets to the bottom and happily runs out the building. No tears today.

I sit for a moment and reflect on what's just taken place and how we got there. I had started by creating a physically safe space, to which I added only the minimum of instruments. I stayed still and watched, responding to whatever Sammy offered us, allowing him to take the lead. I modelled different behaviours for his mum, then encouraged her to take ownership of these. Above all, I paid attention to the little things: the turn of the head, the sideways glance, the roll of the drum, the length of the phrase, and the view from the top of the stairs.

Notes

1. All names and some details have been changed to preserve anonymity.

References

Bowlby, J. (1988). *A Secure Base: Parent-child attachment and healthy human development*. New York: Basic Books.

Harker, E. (2008). Cited in *To Grace the Earth*. UK: Natural Voice Practitioners Network.

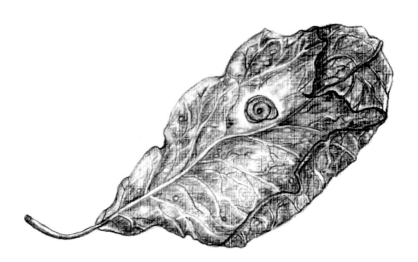

Moments in Music Therapy

Libby Johns

Told by the therapist, *the narrator* and the music.

DEXTER

He throws, he plays, I watch, I listen

I sing, I play, he listens

He sings, I sing, we listen.

~

'You can have the yellow (kazoo) but which colour for Libby?' I ask, while Dexter pulls at the yellow kazoo in my hand. 'Yellow,' Dexter says confirming his preference and dismissing my question. He begins to sounds the kazoo:

'Hoo? Hoo!' It sounds as if he is answering his own vocal question.

The music therapy room was large and long with big bold blue acoustic panels injecting colour to the white walls. The light streamed in from the windows on the far wall and the sound of cars passing by was distant and soft. The shadow of the ti kōuka and harakeke outside created dark shapes on the blue carpet. We were situated in the middle and just off to one side, close to the upright piano positioned against the wall. Three vibrantly coloured gathering drums; large, medium, small, and a slender djembe were clumped opposite the piano. The snare and cymbal were paired and sat ready for action opposite the guitar. Together the instruments formed an uneven square, creating an inner boundary within the perimeter of the room.

Dexter turns to put the kazoo at the bass end of the piano and sits on the stool facing the piano. He strikes the keys as he lets go of the kazoo. It falls to the floor. He directs a statement at his mother, Hannah, which I cannot understand. Dexter begins to explore the piano as Hannah and I sit on the floor watching, waiting to be invited into his musical adventure.

Dexter was a young boy, playful and certain of what he wanted and disliked. Certain sounds and events could become overwhelming for him as he developed his sensory integration and self-regulation skills. It appeared that when Dexter felt out of control he became unsettled and communicated this through rough and aggressive actions and vocalisations reflecting distress and anxiety. He was developing his ability to speak clearly and in short sentences and interact with new people. Dexter spoke mainly to his mother and occasionally to me. His main form of communication in sessions was through physical gestures.

Dexter begins to play rhythmically using both hands simultaneously and independently. He plays cluster chords, whole hands pressing down onto the piano keys:

> Four short lively chords
> with
> descending
> notes in the
> left hand
> followed by a sustained cluster chord.

This feels like a musical statement, finishing one moment and inviting a new moment or possibility. Dexter plays innately, with expectation and anticipation. I jump on the opportunity and match the sustained chord with a vocalisation 'oooooh' … this anacrusis helps me to connect with Dexter's play and further empower it as it becomes the foundation for my singing:

'Piano, piano, piano' pause 'one two three four piano'. The melody jumps and falls then rises, building tension and anticipation.

Dexter joins in on the piano with three ascending individual notes roughly matching the rhythm of my lyrics. As I pause, Dexter slips down off the stool to reposition it, moving closer in and higher up the treble end of the piano. He strikes the piano once more. Does this mean he wants to play more? Is he motivated by my suggestion to play, sing and count? I strum C major on the guitar and respond to his movement. I remind myself to keep it simple, I adjust the tempo, create more space and less texture, reducing the complexity of the harmony.

I was a student music therapist. I had found our seven previous sessions together challenging and was aware that this session needed to be different. I was unsure how Hannah and I could work in a more supportive way. As a student, I felt a self-imposed pressure to deliver, how was I seen? Was I good enough for her child?

I respond, repeating my previous phrase 'piano piano piano' then pause and Dexter begins to play rhythmically on the white keys and count melodically, 'one, two', imitating my lyrical idea. A short pause then Dexter continues 'four, five' and his piano play develops with pitch and rhythm. He is able to coordinate his voice and piano play movements. Dexter has sat and counted at the piano in a previous session but not interacted with me in this way before. I know that Dexter likes counting to five (rather than three or four), so I seek to play with this. Our pulse and metre appear to form naturally as I follow Dexter's last two notes and begin on the <u>strong</u> first beat of the bar.

<pre>
                      five ---' I hold this note,
                four   sliding
                three   down
                  two   with
I count and sing up the scale 'One   my voice.
</pre>

I repeat the same phrase trying to reinforce the pulse, continuity and predictability, with the hope of inviting Dexter to contribute. He does. Our counting song is established. Dexter matches the ascending melody with his piano play and fills in the gap I leave on the third repetition. I sing:

<pre>
                                        'four five.'
                              Dexter sings high
          four' leaving the phrase unfinished and suspended ...
        three
      two
  'One
</pre>

Dexter's 'four' is loud and with exclamation, whilst 'five' is sung quietly in relation. This feels meaningful as Dexter responds constructively and musically to me (an area identified in music therapy for Dexter to develop).

As I considered my clinical notes and the hours of video footage filed, I kept returning to the question 'what made that moment different?' I was drawn to understanding what was happening in the music and soon found that there was more than just notes and sounds to be considered as part of our shared music. These meaningful moments included body language and movement, silence and waiting, eye contact and musical connection. All vital elements to my experience in that moment.

I strum the guitar without singing, helping to give momentum. Dexter responds. My accompaniment acts as an acknowledgement of Dexter's musical contribution; letting his voice be heard over mine.

Four more repetitions of our call and response interaction follow. I count to four and Dexter sings 'five', completing the sequence. Dexter continues to play the piano through this and on the third repeat we are synchronised and begin together with the piano and guitar on the first beat of the bar. As I begin to count for the fourth repetition I count only to the number three, Dexter comes in quickly on the following beat …

'Five'

        'four … four … four' (sings Dexter, he turns to look at me)
        three'
      two
I sing - 'One
reinforced by
his piano play,
co-ordinated
perfectly.

I sing, imitating Dexter's contribution. Our reciprocal play is engaging and energising as we trust and expect each other to contribute.

This also felt like a meaningful moment, as Dexter acknowledged me visually and audibly. This was one of the first moments in our eight sessions that Dexter appeared to truly engage, allow and share his experience with me, intentionally.

We move into a period of free play, engaging with rhythmic elements without a pulse. I attempt to reintroduce the melody after a brief period of silence. 'Oh one, two, three', I pause, Dexter begins to play the piano again and for the next 20 seconds he explores and approaches the piano in five distinctive ways.

First, with both hands almost synchronised as they touch the piano keys. I continue my phrase without guitar accompaniment. Second, Dexter plays a short, followed by a <u>sustained cluster chord</u> using simultaneous hands with intention and articulation as I sing and finish the lyrical phrase: 'Five----' sliding down the scale. Third, Dexter continues this time with:

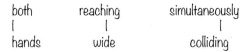

… with the keys as play appears less structured and freer. Dexter appears to increase and decrease the volume as the pitch increases and decreases. I begin again as Dexter plays, I finish the counting sequence at 'four' and pause. Fourth, Dexter plays in the space I leave with two triplet figures, I respond in the space he leaves (albeit brief) '... Fiiiivvvve' repeating, as before. Fifth, Dexter initiates the next phrase with a chord placed high in the treble end of the piano and we play together, synchronised, as I count, stopping once again at 'four'. I pause. Dexter turns around to reference Hannah sitting behind him. As he twists around to the left (away from me) he places his right hand on the keys creating a chord, which appears to function as a signal to break and perhaps stop. We begin a new phase of play. Dexter talks to Hannah and slips off the piano stool to go and meet her. Hannah comes to meet him halfway, they hug and she encourages Dexter to return to the piano.

At the same time I decide it may be time to end this song and count one last time

'One
  two
    three
      four'
        'five.' Dexter completes my phrase singing, on the starting note.

Hannah plays a single key and Dexter responds then moves away to the windchimes, which are placed near the window. Again, Dexter moves away from me. It appears to me that Dexter is initiating 'more' as he begins to play the windchimes, so I follow him with my voice and offer the counting phrase again. Dexter finishes the sequence 'five', in a spoken voice. We repeat once, twice, then Dexter returns to the piano where Hannah is kneeling. Hannah imitates Dexter as she creates sound, singing and playing the piano one key at a time.

Dexter hops up onto her back and leans on the piano to adjust his position; this looks awkward for Hannah but not unfamiliar. The piano is no longer an instrument, rather a noisy object to push off. He finishes the counting sequence for the third time, without the piano, then comes to me requesting the guitar, as he had with the kazoo previously. 'Mine, mine, mine … my turn' Dexter calls. Calmly and slowly I sing the sequence once more, descending, and Dexter completes the phrase with 'five'. His voice is nasal, bright, and urgent. I use a softer timbre in my voice to communicate permission and model gentle negotiating. Hannah offers support saying 'it's Libby's turn', however Dexter continues to pull at the guitar. He appears overwhelmed and in need of a change. I relinquish the guitar,

> 'One
>   two
>   three
>   four
>   five, here you go!'
> I breathe. I wait.

Dexter takes the guitar and begins to explore its sounds. He takes it to Hannah who holds it while Dexter fetches the ukulele. They play together. Hannah is willing to discard her uncertainties about playing the guitar, and explores sounds and the experience of not knowing and creating in the moment with her son.

Dexter and Hannah sit nearby a collection of gathering drums and djembes, and, after listening to their free play, I wonder if our song and interactive play will transfer to this new instrumentation. I approach the drums.

After one minute I reintroduce our song. Perhaps I am still looking for a positive shared ending to what I feel has been a meaningful moment, and subsequently a turning point in our therapeutic process. Dexter and

Hannah play, I add the pulse of the djembe and sing. Dexter responds to the pauses and completes each counting phrase with 'five'. After 40 seconds I change the sequence for the last time and count …

'Five
　　four
　　　　three
　　　　　　two'
(Dexter replies) -　　　'One! … No it's five.'

This clearly punctuates our play and interaction and Dexter makes sure of it by once again removing the instrument from my hands.

As I reflect, this moment felt long and repetitive. However, the pauses, variation in interaction, and simplicity of the melody seemed to create 'newness'. Dexter found an effective way to stop me from continuing to play and was also willing to take small risks during musical interaction to engage with me. It appeared in this interaction that I challenged him and perhaps 'pushed him over his threshold' three times. However, what caught my attention was the developing interaction and duration of parallel and shared play. Dexter began to flow between risk and control:

See–saw
see–Saw
Control–risk
control–Risk
Ground–air–Ground
ground-Air-ground.
How long can we balance together, with our feet in the air?

MAX

A child full of joy and creativity
Waiting to be safe to express
Waiting to be safe to grow
Waiting to be safe to share

~

'Oooohh' I sing. Waiting, anticipating and inviting Max to offer an idea to our shared moment.

We are sitting on the floor holding a beater in each hand. Max waves his in the air. He makes eye contact with me, and begins to strike the floor. Is he acknowledging my invitation to lead, or does he feel safe to initiate and is therefore inviting me to be part of his play? I sing and imitate Max's actions as he transitions from striking the floor to the bongos:

'Copy Max, copy Max, da da da da da ... Be the same, be the same be the same as Max'. The melody is pulsed with jumps and stepwise movement, ascending and descending to create movement and flow.

Sessions took place in a large classroom. The wall heaters on and the video camera off to one side. There were many objects and instruments kept on the periphery of the room, so we created a smaller boundary within the room for our work. We had a large colourful gathering drum, which was on its side, left from our previous activity. There were also many small percussion instruments placed around looking somewhat lost in such a huge room. Like sweets in a lolly scramble, their vibrant and various sounds added colour to our spontaneous play. Occasionally these percussion instruments collided with a foot or other instrument as movement occurred in the room. Max and I sat close to the windows with our beaters, a xylophone and bongo drums each.

Our matching game continues as Max changes to play with one hand, then 'trills' on his bongo drums (alternating between the two drums of the bongos, quickly with his beaters). Max stops. I follow. I use my voice to set up another expectant moment. This time I sustain the note for almost ten seconds, three times longer than the last. Max joins in playing his bongo drums again and initiates slowing the speed of our play. At the same time I fall off the note decreasing in pitch and volume. I join Max briefly on the bongo drums and we finish together quietly. We 'trill' together for three seconds, as if whispering. Max lifts his beaters into the air and I follow. Something is about to change.

Watching and reflecting on this session has given me the opportunity to see many cues and moments of nonverbal communication, which passed by so quickly at the time. As I took time to transcribe just two minutes of live music and interactions to sheet music and text, I was soon able to see and hear more connection in our play then I had previously thought. As we shared a quiet trill together something motivated and encouraged Max to share, initiate and create a new opportunity for me to explore music making with him. When Max lifted his arms and beaters into the air he was ready to lead! This was the first time I felt completely guided by him.

Max begins to play the xylophone; a collection of notes fills the space. He does not appear to have an intention behind his note choices, however his overall phrase (albeit five seconds long) ascends in pitch, as if to ask a question. I join in towards the end of his phrase with a short descending swipe over the xylophone keys. My intention is to create a framework for call and response play, a conversation without words, expressive music making. Max understands and plays three short ascending notes that I imitate. Again Max plays three ascending notes and I imitate him accurately, with rhythm and pitch. And again, this time Max develops his 'call' with a fourth note. I copy. And again, Max extends and creates a long 14-note phrase with rhythmic variation. I copy, this time with my own original phrase. I finish my phrase an octave lower than Max. This feels to me like an answer to his initial question. Max appears to recognise this 'full stop' and begins a new phase of play. He begins to sing! I listen. 'B and D out ... take B and D out and put them, on.' Max sighs and continues to hum briefly:

hum' down and up, soft and contemplative.
'hum   hum
        hum

Max was singing and melodically speaking as he took the B and D keys off the xylophone. This was the first time in our sessions that Max had initiated singing an original song. I had modelled this over the course of our 10 sessions and felt that Max responded well to melodic speech when reinforcing actions, but this took me by surprise.

Max sits with the B and D keys removed from his xylophone:

'Look at my haah ...' Max does not complete the last word of his phrase, instead he looks up to make eye contact with me. I hum three descending notes, encouraging him to continue to weave his way through the music, leading me, trusting that it is safe to venture on.

Max introduces the xylophone again and swipes up along the keys three times ...

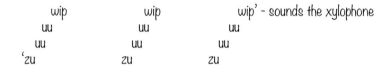

I imitate.

Max goes to play where the B key once sat. He plays rhythmically as his beater strikes the empty space. I imitate. Max looks over to see me copying him. Our rhythmic pulse is loose yet related as I follow Max's lead. Suddenly he slows right down and begins to put his B and D keys back on. I follow immediately and offer vocal reinforcement, 'Oh B and D here they go back on. B for?' I pause for one beat then decide to model by singing 'Butterfly.' I continue, 'and D for?' I pause again and Max responds quickly singing 'Dog'. We make eye contact. It feels like it's now time for me to lead the call and response play and so we sing:

'Oh, what about E? (pause) E for?' I sing as Max locates the E key then looks at me.
'Egg.' Max responds quickly and accurately in the gap.
'Egg.' I repeat, 'E for Egg'.
'E for egg.' Max imitates me vocally and gesturally as we hold our E keys and strike them with our beaters.

'And what aboooout?' I hold and pause on my final note briefly,
'F,' replies Max. We are now sharing the lead and negotiating.
' F, F for?' I sing, suspending the final note. I nod my head, encouraging Max to respond once more.
'Fish.' Max sings.

Max's main challenges were movement and motor-skills oriented and subsequently confidence. Max showed sustained attention to items, objects and activities that interested him. I had often found that Max was not interested or able to engage in verbal conversation, however our nonverbal and vocal interaction showed me that he indeed had the skills required to communicate with ease. It was my desire to foster his confidence in order to generalise these skills, seen in musical interaction, to his social interactions in daily life.

Max and I continue for another six minutes exploring the letters on the xylophone keys and the corresponding words. He is playful, takes small risks, endearing, creative and confident. What a joy it is to be in music, to create meaningful experiences and to empower others to truly just *Be*.

I now understand that these meaningful moments were shared experiences in the co-creation of music, which provided opportunities to foster a responsive interpersonal relationship between the child and therapist. They occurred because the music provided a framework for structure and change through synchronicity, regularity and flow as well as variation, tension, suspension, expectation and anticipation. They were facilitated by musical elements: rhythm, tempo, pitch, melody, harmony, timbre, volume and dynamics; and musical techniques: imitation, pause, space, repetition, anacrusis and gestural actions.

I wanted to know more

I researched

I transcribed

I analysed

I interpreted

I found

I questioned

I wrote

You read

You learn

You experience, if only for a moment …

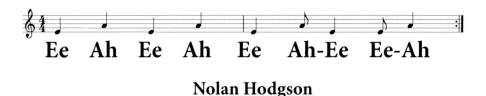

Ee Ah Ee Ah Ee Ah-Ee Ee-Ah

Nolan Hodgson

We are waiting in line, patiently ignoring the chocolate bars and trashy magazines staring at us from the shelves. An equally nutritious selection of pop music and cheesy advertising blares out on a retail radio station overhead. We load our groceries on to the belt where they flow through the dab hands of the cashier and on into a waiting trolley with a sharp *Beep!* from the barcode scanner. Perfunctory conversation is made and we get an insightful glimpse into the diets of those in front of us as their groceries are processed.

Usually I squirm with impatience when forced to stand in line but this time I'm alert and on the job. We're in the supermarket as a class. Four students, one teacher and two teacher aides. We are careful to hold hands with two of the students as we know how tempting those chocolate bars we are surrounded by can be. Another student is busy making conversation with everyone she makes eye contact with while the fourth sits quietly in his wheelchair and, confusingly, is laughing and smiling quietly to himself.

I say confusingly because Joshua is rarely even slightly interested in eating the groceries we buy. Nor do the sumptuous meals that we make from them back at school excite him. In fact we often have to goad him into tasting just a tiny bit after which his face twists inwards like he's bitten into one of those crisp apples that turns out to be rotten and putrid inside.

So his laughter seems all out of place when I notice it here. My confusion is allayed though when the other teacher aide starts chuckling and says 'This is the best part of the supermarket trip, seeing Joshua enjoy all the beeps'.

And that's what it is. The beeps. After hearing this I watch him closely. His smile begins at the corner of his mouth, curving up and slowly spreading across his face as the flow of beeps continues. Those high pitched blasts that snap out from the counter as each item rings through and is added to your bill. Taken collectively, the sounds from every individual checkout combine to form a bizarre chorus of identically-toned beeps, with each counter distinguishable only by the subtle slump in volume from those further away. There is no stable rhythm to it, but any silence is always pregnant with the possibility of one or two or six beeps all dropping simultaneously at any moment. There are also those experienced staff members who can handle a stream of random foodstuffs and process it all through with a steady, reliable pulse.

It is this haphazard ensemble that sets Joshua laughing and smiling. His awareness and appreciation of these environmental sounds was phenomenal and the delight he drew from them severely contagious. In such a cacophonous environment, I tuned out these extraneous noises and saw nothing but a frustrating test of my patience within a sea of tacky advertising and salty consumerism. Yet Joshua was able to tune in, sit back in his wheelchair, and enjoy himself as the beeps rolled in.

We met on my first day of work. Luckily for me, the entire school was going out for a picnic at a local park for the whole day. A teacher introduced me to Joshua and told him I was a musician. He was sitting on a tarpaulin on the ground so I sat down next to him and said hello. He began beating a pulse on the ground with his hand. I joined in and was caught there for most of the day. He gradually began to introduce accents and alter the speed of his playing. Likewise, I began to experiment and his response to changes in tempo and dynamics was fascinating. He could be brought to peals of laughter by accelerations of tempo or sudden shifts in volume. Because of his cerebral palsy, it was difficult for Joshua to maintain a very rapid tempo and he would lose the rhythm completely when he began laughing. I would maintain the rhythm during these faster periods or keep the rhythm going until he regained his composure and joined in again.

After a while, I grew weary of the standard four beats and began introducing offbeats or playing cross rhythms in tandem with his playing. Over time this developed into a couple of short rhythms that we experimented with for over two years and Joshua still remembers these today. Every time I have stopped in to visit his old school I've spent some time with him. As soon as I say hello he will start singing or tapping one of these rhythms we developed and I'll slot back into playing these same little tunes just as I did three years ago.

I worked alongside Joshua over a period of two years. First as a teacher aide in his class and then as a therapy assistant at his school for children with profound and multiple disabilities. There were fewer than twenty students at this school so I was able to spend a significant amount of time enjoying his company and discovering just how much music and sound filled his daily life. Working with Joshua, singing was obligatory. Any conversation involved singing or humming. This did become difficult if we were focusing on maths or fine motor skills but Joshua challenged us to bring music into these areas as well. He was fiercely determined and if we wanted him to engage wholeheartedly, we needed to sing or clap or rhyme or his attention would drift away.

As I was then an aspiring music therapist I always volunteered to accompany students to any music sessions they had. Joshua was a very articulate musician and could play back phrases he'd heard on a keyboard perfectly. Unfortunately fine motor skills were quite difficult for him and so he couldn't play fast or complicated pieces at their usual tempo. He knew exactly how they went however and could sing the intro to Ravel's Boléro or repeat a lengthy Cook Island drumming phrase without getting lost.

While he can speak, both verbally and through a computer, he would always prefer to sing or drum than have a conversation. In my experience, no conversation with Joshua would be complete without some music and often interactions with him are entirely musical. He was adept at using his computer to speak for him but would spend most of his time with this machine pressing buttons rapidly so that the electronic voice couldn't keep up. To compensate it would bleat out a steady stream of gibberish syllables and word segments for long minutes that only Joshua would enjoy.

He is without a doubt the most musical being I have ever encountered, with such a voracious appetite for it that I would say he almost lives and breathes music. I have definitely seen him eat and drink it. He was captivated by toys or instruments that sang or produced sounds and loved spending time with people who would sing and experiment musically with him. Anything that rings or rhymes was popular and he knew all the old nursery rhymes that other people would be familiar with. I'm sure he would have known the alphabet from a very young age. So he might start singing *Row, row row the boat* and wait for you to start singing along with him. Once you joined in he would begin changing the tempo or splicing in and overlaying a different song. Overlapping two distinct rhythms was also hugely entertaining and as soon as you stopped playing he would ask for 'More' or 'More, please' with the 'Please' becoming particularly urgent if he was really enjoying himself.

I always found it very difficult to stop musicking with Joshua as he enjoyed it so much and I find it equally difficult to convey just how big a pull music appeared to have over him. I almost feel that, in his world, music is the sun and rhythm is the gravity that keeps everything else orbiting around it. He attends to his auditory environment with much greater scrutiny than I ever have or probably ever will. He taught me that I can use music in almost any situation and also made me aware of the significance of sound-marks and the ways that sound can define an environment.

We are so involved in the visual world that we are drenched in that we forget to attend to soundscapes. Our brains filter out background noise so we don't notice that buzz the fridge makes or that traffic passing in the background. But there is music in these places. Rhythm and timbre born of unique environments and the ways we interact with them. The only one of these I can recall enjoying before meeting Joshua was in the bathroom of an old block at the college I went to. The urinal was one of those old stalwart sheets of steel built in to the wall, perhaps three metres across and one and a half tall. When in use, this particular urinal had a curious habit in that the entire sheet would distort and pop into a different shape with a satisfying *Bong*, presumably from the change in temperature. While this was fairly disconcerting the first time, it was certainly worth going back for, even if you were in a class on the opposite side of the school. I suppose I enjoyed it for the same reason people enjoy using stairs set up so that each step is a key from a giant keyboard that plays as you walk along it.

A giant keyboard like this was once used to prove the 'fun theory'- the notion that fun is the easiest way to influence people's behaviour and get them walking up stairs rather than taking the escalator. After working with Joshua, I make a particular effort to discover and enjoy these curious auditory artefacts. There is a hill in Aro Valley in Wellington where I can close my eyes and know exactly where I am. The gradient of the ground falls in such a way that it sends hundreds of tiny rivulets of water trickling down through the grass underfoot. On a still night, the sound of these minuscule waterways combine to form the faintest susurration that seems to emanate from everywhere all at once and no one direction in particular. It's as if you are upside down and standing on the tin roof being rained upon, still dry but aware of the moisture all around and singing out to you.

The most recent one I came across while sneezing in a particular spot in the kitchen of my flat. If you stand in line with the fridge on one side and face towards the oven, the echo from this point reverberates back at you from the corners of the room and doesn't appear to decay as fast as the sound does when standing somewhere else. My flatmates and I had a wonderful time shaking all the jars of nuts and grains to see which echo we enjoyed the most, with Brazil nuts and almonds both performing well. I remembered Joshua when I discovered both of these spots, and have gone out of my way to enjoy them both a number of times.

I don't think I enjoy them as much as Joshua appears to enjoy the supermarket or the noises that the horses make which would send him into hysterics while riding a horse at Riding for the Disabled. I am ever thankful that he opened my ears to the existence of these idiosyncratic and entertaining soundscapes that we all inhabit. From the beginning, my friendship with Joshua was built on musical interaction and from then on, Joshua showed me that music and sounds can be squeezed into every single moment possible. Since meeting him I have worked with scores of other people as a music teacher and music therapist. Every one of them has had a unique relationship with music but none as all encompassing as that which I experienced with Joshua. Because of his blindness and cerebral palsy, Joshua was never able to perceive the world visually nor explore it independently in the way that most of us are accustomed to. Instead the world comes to him. While he may never have seen a smile or a sunset, I'm sure his day will begin with birds in the morning, and the subtle shifts in a person's tone of voice when they are happy must be immediately recognisable to him. More significantly though, because of his fondness for and insistence upon interacting through music and rhythm, most of the people in Joshua's world are singing.

Chimes

Marie Willis

A young boy[1]
A mother
A father
A sister
A journey

A diagnosis - a short time
A similar journey traversed before - a sibling
Another journey, this time full of musicking
Chimes: an unknown entity.

A suggestion
A room full of musical instruments
A therapist
A family commitment
An intention - to explore
A wish - to celebrate
Chimes: available.

An assessment
A glance towards shiny silver
An astute mother
A positioning
An invitation
An urge to move - expressed
A supportive hand
A belief
Anticipation
Another ten seconds
A finger movement
An inhale, suspense
A sound
A smile - shared
Chimes: potential.

A response - sung
A stare towards the therapist
A focus
A determination
A mother's encouragement
A decision
Another attempt
A movement - contact
A celebration
Again
Chimes: an opportunity.

Another week
A song about twinkling
A phrase presented
A pause
An effort to move - felt
A ready hand - guided
A sound created
Another phrase - sung
Another movement
A success
Chimes: independence.

A presentation
An audience: care professionals, caring
A video
A witnessing
A collective gasp
A collective agreement
An idea acted on
A purchase
A gift - for home
Chimes: available 24/7.

Another month
A song repeated
A phrase sung
A pause created
A readiness
An absence of delay - immediate response
Another phrase added
An action - perfectly timed, anticipated
A joint venture
Chimes: a meaningful shared experience.

A guitar
An eagerness to reach
An opportunity to expand
A repertoire building
A supportive father keen to accompany
A new instrument - glockenspiel
A learning curve
A tune mastered
Chimes: integral.

An attentive sister, aspiring
A dream - to play guitar
A challenge
A perseverance
A joy
A brother, an audience
Awake or asleep
Chimes: unquestionably incorporated.

A period of growth
A joyful journey
Affirmation coloured by humour
An exploration of communicative possibilities
Chimes: a consistent preference.

A scare
A period in hospital
A welcome onto the ward
A session or two with aunties, grandmas, cousins
An ocean drum - accessible
An ocarina - admired
A sitting with the unknown
Chimes: acknowledged.

A recovery
A shift in sessions - at home
An uncertainty - queried
A decision to continue
A contribution - valued
Chimes: ever present.

A birthday,
Another year!
A celebration
A ride in a fire truck - asleep!
A gift - a prayer
A photo
A cake
A party
Chimes: the cousins' curiosity.

A period of sleepiness - weeks
Apprehension - how long?
Answers - ambiguous
Chimes: a comfort.

A continuation
A mother and father inspired
An eagerness to learn
Attention turned to learning tunes, percussion - tuned
Chimes: a constant.

A phone call
An inhale
An exhale
A sigh - some relief
Chimes: silent.

A request - to play
A ceremony - to celebrate
A song repertoire shared
A favourite story read aloud
A remembering
An acknowledgement of strengths
An expression of gratitude
Chimes: a story-telling motif.

A family grieving
A closure accepted
A remembrance
A space to laugh, to cry
A time to reflect and to look forward
Chimes: recalled.

A memory shared of a cessation of breath
A giving of breath
A moment of silence
A mother's love
A song about twinkling - sung
Another breath taken
Another three hours - shared
A time for final goodbyes.

Chimes: a reminder of the power of music to inspire, to invite, to ignite,
to motivate, to animate, to encourage, to bond, to express,
to carry, to comfort, to unite, to hold.

~

Notes
1. Shared with the kind permission of T's family.

Learning to Play: Together

Marie Willis

Prologue

Let's both go for a walk today, walking hand in hand,
Walking tall, no cares at all, together strong, we stand.

Let's both go for a walk today, walking by and by,
just now you were beside me and suddenly I heard you cry ...

Here we are, down a hole, how did we get here?
We fe.....ll down, we fe.....ll down, down 'til we landed here.

How do we get out again? I think I need your help my friend,
Reach out your hand and help me stand,
together we will climb again.

This story charts the process of transformation for a young boy called
Edward[1] who has autism. It illustrates the changes that came about within
his family dynamic as they learned to be playful and to play together.
Although goals relating to communication and social behaviour were
formulated with his parents and informed the work, it is the course that

Edward steered for himself that is the focus of this narrative; that of teaching his parents to develop their play skills with him. Edward's parents have given verbal consent for the case to be presented in public forums. Names and some details have been changed to protect confidentiality.

Beginning (Sessions 1-7)

Edward's arrival was announced by a brisk march into the building, and a slam of the waiting room door behind him, shutting Mum outside, and ensuring that I knew he was most certainly inside. I went to greet him and found him hiding his face behind a book cover. My cheery 'hello' was met with silence, and a motionless body. As I waited, two eyes peeped out from the hiding place and I sensed his invitation to 'find me'.

When Edward and I first began to work together, the theme of control characterised his use of the music therapy relationship and frustration was evident in his aggression towards me and his parents, particularly his mother. Yet, within his apparently controlling and hostile behaviour I began to observe a strong desire to connect; to engage in playful and reciprocal social interaction. As our sessions progressed it became clear that he was urging me to share his motivation to play beyond the therapy room to include his parents. I gave much thought to the best way of approaching this task with relation to the family cultural dynamic, however it was Edward who ultimately steered the way and beckoned his parents to playfully enter his world with the theme of 'being found' pervading the course of our music therapy sessions and coming to symbolise the essence of the work.

The music therapy room was small and windowless. As I witnessed Edward's drumming I felt shut out. He moved his arms in a chaotic yet deliberate thrashing motion, creating a near-deafening torrent of sound. I attempted to connect musically, but my instrumental and vocal sounds were drowned out. I felt a sense of wonder at the intensity of Edward's playing, and I was reminded of my role to wait and endure, comforted by the knowledge that the student music therapist who had previously worked with Edward had experienced similar feelings of redundancy.[2]

Edward's drumming would continue for up to 20 minutes at the beginning of each session, after which he showed interest in exploring the other available instruments. All instruments, that is, except the piano which he refused to play. He usually frowned when I sought to play it, or commented with cross or disappointed inflection: 'What you doing?' Edward's mum had been a singer and a music teacher in East Asia before she and her husband moved to New Zealand with Edward and his brother. She was keen for Edward to learn to play the piano. Early on in the work I found myself wondering whether for Edward the piano symbolised a difficult relationship with his mum, and one he would rather leave firmly outside the therapy door.

Edward frequently ignored my suggestions of what, or how we might play in our first sessions. Underneath his stubborn refusal however, I sensed a keenness to explore, and a willingness for me to be involved in such exploration. Internally, I adopted a stance of curiosity as I continued to offer ideas for shared musical play, presented with a beckoning and playful voice.

Whilst use of the drums seemed reserved for the initial release and expression of loud chaotic feelings, the wind instruments became our means of conversation and dialogue. In one of the early assessment sessions a sequence developed whereby one of us would make a stream of highly expressive vocal sounds into the bell of the horn, punctuated with either a horn or kazoo blast to finish. Meanwhile, the other person listened, the horn held to their ear like a hearing trumpet or telephone. Edward readily engaged in these interactive exchanges and repeatedly initiated them in early sessions. Over time his contributions grew increasingly elaborate and creative.

After these playful interactions, it was hard for him to leave the room at the end of sessions. I wondered why it was so difficult for him to leave and, without placing any particular expectations on the ending, I waited for his communication to reveal itself. At the end of session five, Edward asked for his mum to collect him. From this point forth in our work, the ritual of being 'found' at the end of sessions became a significant element towards helping Edward's parents to literally and metaphorically 'meet' Edward through playful interaction.

During the process of reviewing the assessment period with Edward's parents and through attending a meeting about his progress at school, it became apparent that family members and school staff were sometimes perplexed about how to engage and interact with him. There was support for music therapy however, and so our journey continued.

Middle Period (Sessions 8-43)
Being found and being woken

> *The end of the session was approaching and Edward lay on the bean bag. 'Get Mum!' barked Edward whilst he busied himself covering every inch of his body with the cream cloth. I was reminded of the way Edward hid when I greeted him in the waiting room and wondered if he was requesting to be found by his parents in the same way that he invited me to find him at the start of our sessions?*

Many sessions occurred during which I fetched either parent to help Edward leave the room. I sensed some disappointment or disapproval from his parents that such intervention was required and they did not initially realise the invitation to play. For weeks I extensively modelled: 'One, two, three … wake up Edward!' as I pulled away the cloth to reveal an expressionless Edward underneath. At first Dad engaged with this interaction more readily than Mum. During one session he spontaneously struck up a drum roll on the congas before he pulled away the cloth. Edward smiled warmly in response and requested that this musical prologue should be sounded whenever Dad collected him. Mum, on the other hand, seemed unwilling to engage in such a playful manner. She commonly stood over Edward with her arms folded and wore a frown upon her face, whilst scolding him in Chinese or English. It seemed to me that she perceived a 'naughty' or non-compliant child rather than an opportunity to connect through play.

The weeks progressed and Edward's levels of responsiveness and reciprocity within sessions increased. Our musical engagements became more playful with frequent turn-taking exchanges and imaginative play. However, when confronted with the stand-off which occurred when Mum was asked to find Edward, I became aware of how these achievements became suddenly lost, the fun extinguished. The stand-off was expressed in the motionless bodies and expressionless faces of both parties once the cloth had been removed. Sometimes, at such junctures, Edward would look expectantly from me to Mum, and back to me. I soon realised that he was imploring me to help teach his parents how to engage, find, wake and play with him.

One day I decided to adopt the routine of stepping out of the room to allow Mum or Dad and Edward space to work out the transition together. Raising Edward to his feet still continued to be a struggle however so I stepped back into the engagement and added an extra aspect to the routine; that of reaching out a hand to help pull Edward to his feet whilst encouraging Mum or Dad to do the same. I frequently found myself saying to Edward's parents 'It's okay', referring to Edward's need to be met in this way. At the end of one session I was moved when Edward himself turned to Mum and said in a reassuring tone like mine 'It's okay'. At the end of our 12th session Mum managed a smile. The usually tense dynamic was immediately broken and Edward responded by jumping up and giving first me and then Mum a hug.

The musical conversations that took place in the early sessions with the aid of accessible wind instruments, laid the way for exploration of a variety of vocal sounds which were often presented by Edward in this next period of our journey together. The snores, sighs and yawns which playfully emerged in our exchanges instigated exploration of the themes of sleeping and hiding. These games invariably involved Edward lying down and covering himself with the cloth whilst expressing an assortment of grunts, snorts and snores. A song developed which I called 'A very funny shape'. The title referred to the 'very funny shape' made by Edward's limbs as he lay under the cloth. I gradually named the lumps as knees, shoulders and elbows before the song culminated in a pulling back of the cloth to reveal Edward's face: ' … I see two knees, two elbows and shoulders … it must be Edward!'

The theme of hiding was prevalent throughout the work, manifesting in a number of other engagements between Edward and myself, and between Edward and his parents. Susan Linn comments: 'Those endless games of peek-a-boo are actually manifestations of early grappling with a lifetime of departures and arrivals, of comings and goings, and about testing a newly formed understanding that people and objects exist even when they are out of sight' (2008, p.15).

This seemed to be the case for Edward. In my own supervision I was helped to reflect that extensive repetition and revision of hide-and-seek play in particular was a common theme of any child's development. It seemed evident that Edward had a strong need to revisit the concept of 'hiding' and of being 'found' again and again, and was taking the opportunity within music therapy sessions to practise this social engagement with me and his family.

In an attempt to utilise the instruments in the room, whilst at the same time working on the concepts 'inside', 'on top of', 'underneath' and 'behind' to reinforce Edward's speech and language therapy goals, I introduced a new variation of the game, hide-and-seek. Using the broken seventh chord melody from the song 'Mr Mistoffelees' (from the musical 'CATS') to build suspense, I slowly sang: 'Is he under the cymbal? ... No! ... Is he on top of the drum? ... No! ... Is he behind the piano? ... No! Then where can he be? ... Boo! I've found you!'

Edward repeatedly requested this game during the middle period of our work. Initially he would order me to 'find' him again and again, but over time he came to enjoy being the 'finder' too. Each time he played this role, his voice grew more expressive as he sought to closely imitate my words and vocal inflections. Gradually a more colourful palette of emotional nuances became shared.

At the end of our 34th session, Edward requested a 'Wake up song'. Suspecting that he was recalling a song from his previous episode of therapy with the student music therapist, I said that Mum and I would need his help with this song. I invited Mum to our room and created a simple song, incorporating a tune Edward had hummed. The first three phrases of the song were accompanied by tickling motions on Edward's stomach and limbs as he lay covered by the cloth. Sometimes he showed his eyes from underneath the cloth, sometimes, his whole face. On the fourth and final phrase of the song, the cloth was playfully whisked away and Edward was encouraged to stand and exit the room. We continued to use this song each week until sessions ended. The inclusion of tickling gestures heightened the playful nature of the interaction by way of arousing Edward's anticipation, which in time served to break his stony gaze towards Mum and I, offering instead a smile. Over time I was encouraged to observe Mum gradually engaging in a more playful manner, and to witness the affection Edward showed her in response.

Dialogues

The repetitious and somewhat exaggerated vocal and visual modelling I expressed each week had, it seemed, assisted advances in Edward's use of speech, as well as enhancing his general communication skills. Like many people on the autism spectrum, Edward responded well to visual gestures and to emotive tones of voice and dynamic body gesturing. The wind instrument dialogues described earlier were a sonic equivalent, creating a pantomime-like exchange between us consisting primarily of grunts and expressions of surprise and fatigue.

While Edward's mum on occasion commented with dismay about Edward's inappropriate sudden screeches at home and in public places, the new sound that literally exploded one day within the therapy room was that of the sneeze. Sneezes, along with comments about smells, soon replaced the initial gestures of surprise and fatigue. Sneezes, we learned came in all shapes and sizes! In one session the simple gesture of a sneeze was explored at great length when Edward initiated a conversation about noses and smells. With a tone of curiosity in his voice Edward engaged my attention with a question: 'Do you smell?' My response was a playful recitative-like monologue incorporating the words: 'itchy nose', 'twitch', 'sniff' and 'wiff'.

Clearly, these words and my accompanying dramatic gestures appealed to Edward who promptly began to copy me, sniffing the air and the instruments around him. As sniffing and twitching gestures gathered momentum I slipped over to the piano and struck up a harmonic framework. I felt the opportunity for a song. Edward, who as I mentioned earlier, disliked me playing the piano, immediately questioned, in a sharp tone of voice, what I was doing. However, he was sufficiently caught up in our evolving story line to express any further protest. For the next six minutes we engaged in the co-creation of an improvised song about sneezing. The song was richly peppered with sneezes of all kinds, including exaggerated 'Aaaaaaahhh-ccchooooos'.

This song was one of our most creative and co-operative ventures, and one of the few times that Edward tolerated my playing at the piano, to the extent that our sing-song voices cadenced together after a rousing music-hall-type finale! Every time I have subsequently viewed those six minutes on the video recording, I find myself smiling with surprise and delight at what was achieved that day. Edward's receptivity and apparently irresistible desire to sustain reciprocal play, initiated acceptance of an instrument that he had previously treated with disdain. A musical bridge was established which facilitated ongoing affective co-creation and shared meaning-making.

Falling

In session 32, Edward introduced a new theme, that of falling. At the end of our last game of hide-and-seek towards the end of the session, Edward promptly pretended to fall, and laid himself face-down upon the floor. He then instructed me to get down on the floor beside him. Together we pretended to climb up out of the 'hole' we had apparently found ourselves in. Repeatedly, just before we reached the top, Edward mimed falling back down again, often reaching out to clasp my arm, pulling me down with him. After several 'falls', and unsure how to proceed, I decided to sing our goodbye song whilst keeping my voice upbeat, and encouraged Edward to climb up out of the hole. To my surprise, Edward followed me jogging out of the music room to the waiting room, where *he* 'found' Mum who had clearly heard us coming and had playfully hidden behind her magazine. What a role reversal! I thought.

In the session that followed, Edward initiated the falling theme once again. I played a falling gesture on the piano at which point Edward took me by the arm saying: 'All together now.' We mimed falling down and climbing up together, complete with sounds of exclamation as we fell.

Initially, my thoughts surrounding the theme of falling down a hole were: 'This is not good, for both the client and the therapist to be at the bottom of a hole together!' Shortly, however, I realised that Edward was inviting me to be there *with him*, and I came to see the opportunity for play, exploration and discovery. I decided that this play scenario could provide opportunity for fostering Edward's growing sense of independence, of self-control and confidence. The following two song excerpts, improvised in the moment, helped frame the initial scenarios Edward presented, and were subsequently revisited many times in future sessions:

Going For A Walk
Marie Willis

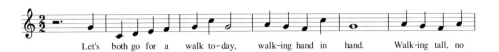

Let's both go for a walk to-day, walk-ing hand in hand. Walk-ing tall, no

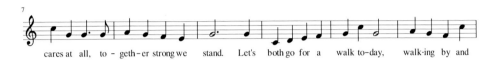

cares at all, to - geth-er strong we stand. Let's both go for a walk to-day, walk-ing by and

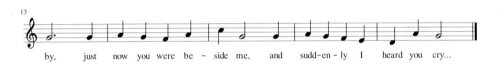

by, just now you were be - side me, and sudd-en - ly I heard you cry...

Down A Hole
Marie Willis

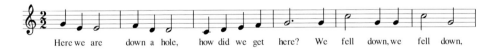

Here we are down a hole, how did we get here? We fell down, we fell down,

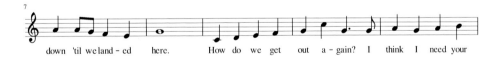

down 'til we land - ed here. How do we get out a - gain? I think I need your

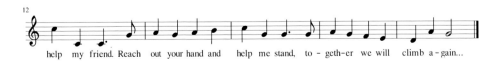

help my friend. Reach out your hand and help me stand, to - geth-er we will climb a-gain...

Over the next few weeks we repeatedly practised falling down and working together to climb back up. I held in mind the possible symbolism of this play; of helping Edward to 'stand on his own two feet', to be able to think and act for himself, and to master his own rescue. Over time our role-play progressed from climbing up side by side, to me climbing up and reaching a hand down to Edward, to me staying at the top of the hole and sending an imaginary rope down to aid his climb, and finally, to simply verbally encouraging him to use his own hands, feet and strength to climb up by himself.

Each time Edward and I engaged in the above journey I was reminded of the following poem by Portia Nelson (2012):

Autobiography in Five Short Chapters[3]

I   I walk down the street.
There is a deep hole in the sidewalk.
I fall in.
I am lost … I am helpless.
It isn't my fault.
It takes forever to find a way out.

II I walk down the same street.
There is a deep hole in the sidewalk.
I pretend I don't see it.
I fall in again.
I can't believe I am in the same place.
But it isn't my fault.
It still takes a long time to get out.

III I walk down the same street.
There is a deep hole in the sidewalk.
I see it is there.
I still fall in … it's a habit.
My eyes are open.
I know where I am.
It is my fault.
I get out immediately.

IV I walk down the same street.
There is a deep hole in the sidewalk.
I walk around it.

V I walk down another street.

Nelson's poem resonated with this period of the work for me because of its theme of empowerment. Empowerment that arises when we take action to prevent ourselves from repeating the same habitual patterns, and succeed in creating new pathways.

A few weeks prior to a meeting to review our work, I began discussing my thoughts with Edward's mum regarding ending therapy as Edward was consistently demonstrating achievement in the agreed goals. In the review meeting I stressed to Edward's parents the effort Edward had exerted in order to achieve these goals. I also sought to highlight how influential his motivation for social engagement had been to these developments and how significant their own willingness to engage playfully with him had been in the process. Edward was present in this meeting. He enthusiastically took charge of working the remote control to show his parents the video footage I had selected to highlight the extent of our musical playfulness.

It was important that Edward was part of this meeting as I wanted him to hear, in front of his parents, my recognition of the work he had done, and perhaps for him to hear this reflected back in their responses. His parents commented that they still felt challenged by Edward's behaviour in the home environment, however, they acknowledged that significant progress in several areas had been made within the music therapy setting. It was agreed that we would work towards an ending of music therapy.

Edward's parents informed me that arrangements had recently been made for him to receive piano instruction. Until this meeting, I had wondered whether the drive to commence piano lessons was motivated by Edward's desire or his mum's. I had expressed concerns about this and also wondered how Edward would manage the very different musical relationship and expectations in music lessons. Related to the former point, I was trepidatious that all the work carried out in the music therapy room that had helped to forge a more playful interactional style, may be rapidly undone if Edward felt pushed into learning the piano. However, on preparing for the review meeting and the ending of therapy I came to recognise Edward's readiness, from the perspective of both social and musical skills, to engage in a teacher-student relationship.

Ending (Sessions 44-49)

> *'Monster, angry monster', communicated Edward in a gruff voice whilst puffing out his chest and arms into a humanoid shape that triggered from the recesses of my mind an image of the 'Incredible Hulk'. 'Warrior', he added, motioning towards me. Somewhat taken aback by this new theme in our relationship, I hesitated ... and then reached for an instrument. Edward blocked my path, making it clear that instruments were not to be used in this new play engagement. I suddenly felt paralysed at the thought of having to respond without the intermediary of a musical instrument at my fingertips. Acting was not my strong point. 'Golly!' I thought, 'I'm not a play therapist, I'm a music therapist, surely there should be music somewhere in the session?'*

Whilst there was a re-visiting of many of our familiar musical interactions during our last sessions, Edward surprised me each week by presenting new play ideas including a role play about an angry monster who lived down a hole and was fought by a skilled warrior. While ruminating on my concerns about the sudden absence of music in our sessions and Edward's demands for me to theatrically embody an archetypal character, I recalled a music therapy paper by Steve Cobbett. Cobbett (2007) describes how music and other media used within a therapeutic relationship have the capacity to be utilised as a form of symbolic communication. He speaks of the use of role play in his work with children and adolescents with emotional and behavioural difficulties as seeming 'useful in that the children were often physically enacting important narratives in their lives and experimenting with different roles and solutions' (p.4).

Edward's mum's perspective on the arrival of the 'monster' in the therapy room was that Edward was referencing an animation character from a television program. I explained that perhaps Edward's introduction of a monster character provided another safe or distanced means for him to express, represent and /or reference anger and frustration; anger and frustration he once expressed through loud, chaotic drumming. I found myself reflecting on the possible significance of Edward's introduction of an opposing character (the warrior) alongside the 'angry monster' at this juncture; the ending of our journey together.

At first Edward wanted solely to play the role of the monster, and requested that I play the role of the warrior. Over time, he more frequently directed me to play the monster whilst he delighted in playing the skilled warrior. I was encouraged by Edward's experimentation; his willingness to 'play' with a new way of being, exploring the role of someone who had mastered particular skills in order to survive in the face of adversity. The power and importance of pretend play is eloquently expressed by Linn:

> Pretend play combines two wondrous and uniquely human characteristics - the capacity for fantasy and the capacity for, and need to, make meaning of our experience. By fantasy I mean imagination, daydreams and the stories we may or may not share with others that design the future, reshape the past, make new things possible, and illustrate powerful feelings. By making meaning, I mean the drive to reflect on and wrestle with information and events so that they make sense to us, enrich us, and help us gain a sense of mastery over our life experience (2008, p.12).

I was surprised and delighted by Edward's capacity for such imaginary play. His interest in new musical and other play ventures was not confined to the music therapy sessions. After one of our final sessions, Mum informed me with clear joy and excitement that she and Edward had been spending a few minutes each day engaged in musical learning. Edward had been learning to sing and play *Twinkle twinkle little star* using solfège musical names and chord buttons on a toy guitar, and had recently asked to transfer this tune onto the piano.

Towards the end of Edward's attendance at the music therapy centre, colleagues and I frequently noted the positive changes in Edward's general presentation, his mum's brighter disposition and the more amenable relationship between them. A short while after the end of Edward's sessions, I arranged a meeting with his mum to follow up and to discuss her perspective regarding the impact of music therapy for Edward and family life. At the meeting I suggested that the progressions Edward had made in every sphere of his life had been impacted simultaneously by the input from school staff and therapists, by the extra-curricular activities he participated in, and by her and her husband's own commitment to his development.

I learned that she had kept a diary since Edward was born. In our meeting she shared with me some of the positive progress Edward had made recently, both in terms of his academic and social skills development. I was most encouraged to hear that she perceived Edward to be engaging in more conversational dialogue and expressing genuine empathic interest in family members. She shared poignant anecdotes describing how Edward had demonstrated concern and affection towards her, and had managed to participate meaningfully in humorous family interactions. She commented, with a smile, that Edward was showing increased interest in what others did. I was moved to hear that Edward's brother was showing greater interest in return and was helping him with his homework.

When I enquired about Edward's parents' hopes for his future, his mum referenced the strong East Asian work ethic that influenced her and her husband's approach to rearing their children. She recognised that her initial hopes for Edward to attend university may be a dream but she maintained her hope that he would continue to develop his musical skills. When I asked how Edward was engaging with his piano lessons she said: 'To me, like a normal child learning music, not a child with autism'.

The Onward Journey

'Our greatest glory consists not in never falling, but in rising each time we fall' Ralph Waldo Emerson.

> *Near the start of our final session, Edward pointed to an imaginary hole on the floor and said, 'Walk around!' After engaging in pointedly walking around the hole for several minutes, Edward suddenly 'fell in' … but not into a hole, into 'water', he informed me. I asked if he could swim. 'No!' came his reply as he indicated he needed help. I threw an imaginary rope into the water which he took hold of, pulled himself to the 'shore' and climbed out.*

Providing models and opportunities to 'play' within a consistent safe relationship and space enabled Edward to develop familiarity with 'falling down holes' and wrestling with the 'monsters' in his life. These experiences also afforded him the opportunity to experiment with alternative scenarios and outcomes, developing self-confidence and honing his skills as a 'warrior' in the process. On reflection, it appeared that Edward had learnt not necessarily to fear or avoid the 'holes in the road' rather, to endeavour to find ways to climb his way out of them.

After our final session I once again found myself reflecting on Nelson's poem. It seemed that Edward and his family were more frequently able to side-step habitual patterns of behaviour and interaction, and were demonstrating that they knew how to engage in more empowering interpersonal exchanges. Edward's days of music therapy were over and he was 'walking down a different street', one where his social and musical interests were being met; one where he and his family were, musically and otherwise, able to share and play together.

Notes

1. Edward's story has previously been presented at a Music Therapy New Zealand conference (Bagley, 2008).
2. The work presented here took place at the Raukatauri Music Therapy Centre, Auckland over a fourteen month period of individual work and builds upon ten months of previous work with a music therapy student on placement at the Centre.
3. Copyright © 1993, by Portia Nelson from the book There's A Hole in My Sidewalk. Reproduced with kind permission from Beyond Words Publishing, Hillsboro, Oregon.

References

Bagley, M. (2008) *Learning to play: Together*. Music Therapy New Zealand Annual Conference 'Making sound progress through cultural diversity, Tikanga-a-iwi; He ara pai, he ara pūoru', Rotorua, New Zealand.

Cobbett, S. (2007). Playing at the boundaries: Combining music therapy work with other creative therapies in individual work with children with emotional and behavioural difficulties. *British Journal of Music Therapy*, *21*(1): 3-11.

Linn, S. (2008). *The case for make believe: Saving play in a commercialized world*. New York: The New Press.

Nelson, P. (2012). *There's a hole in my sidewalk: The romance of self-discovery*. New York: Atria Books/Beyond Words Publishing Inc.

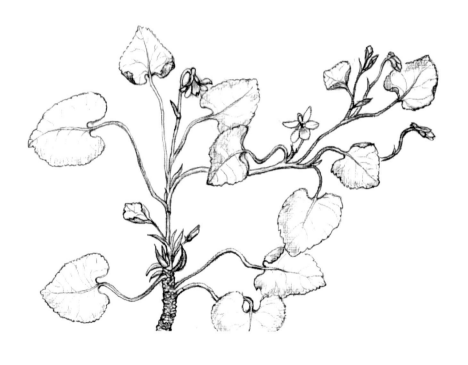

Only Connect

Claire Molyneux

When I was about 16 years old, a teacher gave me a framed print – a picture by Rosina Wachtmeister of a piano and a cello. On the back, the teacher had written the words *Only connect* which he attributed to the author E.M. Forster. I used to wonder what this phrase meant and why my teacher might have chosen it. I have since read the novel *Howards End* from which the phrase comes: 'Only connect the prose and the passion, and both will be exalted and human love will be seen at its highest. Live in fragments no longer.' And still I do not really understand why the teacher chose those words. I like to think that he had some insight into the career path I would eventually choose, that of working as a music therapist. Nearly 30 years later and reflecting on many years of building relationships through the work of music therapy, I hold those two words central to each encounter: only connect.

And so, I wondered how I was going to connect with the beautiful, rather ethereal young woman I found myself sitting opposite. She was small with the most intense dark eyes and long dark hair, her left hand resting on her lap, her right hand guarded and held close to her body, still recovering from a fracture a year earlier. Her body, twisted, resting in a wheelchair and her small feet poking out from under a long lilac skirt. Her mother said she liked piano music, that she used to dance with her hands and smile, but that she seemed rather depressed at the moment. Her mother said she could communicate with her eyes and that sometimes she spoke. And still, I wondered, how could we connect? What could I say or play that would build a bridge between our worlds? Her name was Mali and our first meeting had such a profound effect on me that I spoke about it with my supervisor. As I told the story, my supervisor shared her image of a bird with a broken wing. Not only a broken wing I thought, but a broken voice too.

The guitar was our first bridge, forming a connection between my body and hers. Mali reached out with her left hand, feeling the vibration on the body of the guitar. Later, she would pluck the strings as she danced with her fingers to my voice. Mali came to know and anticipate our greeting song and sometimes when she arrived sleepy, she would rouse and smile as I sang. We settled into a fairly predictable routine of weekly music therapy sessions. We usually started with the guitar, a tentative greeting song: Mali still, listening; me inviting, watching, waiting for a cue that what I was offering was okay and might elicit a response. The greeting song would give way to some improvisation on the guitar and from this I could be guided by Mali's responses to an understanding of her feeling state. Thus together we journeyed through each session, with the music guiding and framing our experiences.

I sometimes wondered how I really knew what to play with Mali. We had a greeting song, but sometimes the greatest connection was in the open strings of the guitar which I played to match her breathing. I looked to Mali for signs of when to stop and when to continue and I found them in her almost imperceptible sighs, her frowns, smiles and eventually her vocalisations.

As we got to know each other, her mother and carer told me they felt her depression was lifting. They felt she was discovering how to feel joy and pleasure again. As Mali began to show herself to me, I learned that she did indeed dance with her hands to the music I played, she blinked with both eyes to let me know when something felt or sounded right or she wanted more, and gradually she found the guitar and the windchimes with her fingers, and rested her hand on the piano as I played.

One week, we were sitting next to each other at the piano, Mali in her wheelchair, me on the piano stool. She reached and took my hand, holding on tightly as I continued to play. My fingers searched the piano for the notes that would speak of the connection that now existed between us and as they did so, I found myself playing a familiar melody: the opening phrase of *Scarlet Ribbons*. I played the phrase a second time, questioning whether this was indeed where my fingers should be. Mali smiled and shuddered. She knew this song and seemed pleased that I had 'got there.' I have often wondered how the song made itself known between us. It is a song from my childhood, poised and held in my relationship with my mother and, as I was to find out after the session, was also a song that held a special place in the maternal line between Mali, her mother and grandmother. I played the song often in our sessions, exploring the connection it created between us and wondering at the eloquence of Mali's subtle communication and responses.

I looked forward to our weekly sessions which had found an easy flow, a rhythm, as I moved from guitar to oboe, drum and voice to piano, and Mali listened and responded with her hands dancing, her voice and her breath. As I played, I observed Mali, watching her face, feeling the rise and fall of her breath, listening for the quiet, almost inaudible vocal sounds. In this way, the connection and communication between us deepened. And so, when in one session the flow felt clunky, something was out of place, the connections faltering; I knew I needed to listen more deeply. I focused on Mali's breathing and played the piano to match her pulse. The music that grew from this was slow, minor in key. It was very hard to match Mali's breath and as I persisted, I became aware of a strong experience of grief. Our music had expressed pain, grief and confusion before but not like this. I wondered whose the grief was and what place it had in our work together. At the end of the session, I shared with Mali's mother this information. Immediately she explained that they had just heard of the death of a close family friend and were grieving this loss. Again I was struck by the powerful way in which Mali was able to express and communicate her feelings. I was reminded of a conversation I had with Clive Robbins who talked about the importance of letting our clients teach us. Mali was teaching me to listen even more deeply and to trust that in listening deeply, we would be able to connect.

Mali and I worked together for nearly three years. For several months, her mother and carer joined the sessions. At times, Mali and I seemed to be creating music for the whole group, building and honouring the strong connections that existed between us as women. At other times, it was important to protect the space for Mali on her own, to allow us both to fully experience the musical moment without additional demands or expectations from her mother or carer. Our music therapy journey came to an end as other demands took my time to different places and Mali transitioned to a new therapist.

Mali, who had lived gracefully with multiple and complex disabilities, died in July 2010. When I heard, I was deeply shocked. How could she be gone? How would her family learn to live without her? I felt guilty that I had not been as present for her in the 18 months since our sessions had finished, that I had let the connection we had experienced slip as the demands of my own busy work and family life took precedence. And yet the connection we had established was still there and now shared and held by two other music therapists who had worked with Mali, both of whom I had the privilege of supervising.

When I heard of her death, I visited the family home where Mali was waiting to be buried, her small body lying on soft blankets and supported by pillows, lilac and purple ribbons leading the way. And there, as I played *Scarlet Ribbons* on her grandmother's piano, I gratefully wept at the privilege of knowing this young woman.

Mali's mother asked me to help with some music for Mali's funeral. She said Mali wanted a 'life party'; not a funeral but a celebration with music and dancing. I was faced with a dilemma: how to honour Mali's life and the relationship I had with her and her family, and how to respect the family's wishes. Was it appropriate for me to play? What would I play, could I even play? The family had a clear idea of two songs they wanted to sing and her mother explained that she felt sure I would know what else was needed. The songs I could provide, it was the *what else* that I was less sure about.

Guided by the family, myself and two other music therapists played the songs that were requested and then two of us improvised at the piano. This was really the only way we knew to connect with Mali's family and friends, in the way we had connected with Mali. As we played, I focused on listening to and feeling what was happening in the room. As the piano music soared, the children started to dance around Mali's open casket, waving ribbons and smiling, touching Mali. In her death, Mali could truly be free, free to move and dance, no longer a bird with a broken wing, but a beautiful, soaring bird, free to fly and sing. Sharing and celebrating Mali's life through music was the greatest thing we could offer in that moment and the most fitting way to honour and connect with her life.

Florence

Alison Talmage

I had the pleasure of knowing Florence towards the end of her fulfilling life as wife, mother, grandmother and teacher. A life lived in Canada and then New Zealand, with family nearby and overseas. A love of music enriched Florence's life; playing the piano from childhood, singing in church, learning the violin alongside her own children, treating them to symphony concerts. She continued to sing, play and listen to music in her later years when she developed Alzheimer's disease, in which dementia symptoms progressively affect a person's memory, thinking, language and their capacity to perform everyday tasks.

I met Florence when her family encouraged her to participate in music therapy experiences.[1] Florence, supported by her daughter Louise, joined a therapeutic choir as a means of sustaining her musical interests and social connectedness. The CeleBRation Choir[2], an initiative of the Centre for Brain Research, is a singing group for people living with neurological conditions. We know that people with dementia often continue to enjoy and respond to music, and Florence's family hoped that music therapy would sustain her musical skills and offer opportunities to meet and connect with other people. The choir's repertoire encompassed familiar folk songs, Broadway tunes, hits from past decades, and seasonal songs for Christmas and Anzac Day.

When we meet, I am struck by Florence's bright smile, her slight puzzlement about the unfamiliar surroundings and her acceptance of the warm support offered by her daughter. Florence sings when the songs are familiar. Blending her voice with others, her spontaneous harmonies enrich the choral sound. She listens and smiles when she doesn't recognise the song. Like most of us, she favours songs remembered from the past, the strong emotions of adolescence and early adulthood establishing our musical preferences.

As an open group, the choir welcomed other family members who came occasionally: Florence's husband, Fred; a granddaughter; and Fred's sister, visiting from overseas. Although Florence could not fully express her experience of belonging to this group, her apparent enjoyment resonates with reflections of other participants.

It's lovely just to sit there singing away too, and just to look around and watch everybody participating at their own level, in their own way, with no pressure. They don't have to do ten of those or eight of those. They're just singing or they're not singing, or they're singing that bit and not that bit. And it's such a level playing field. It's a joy to behold, honestly (Carer of a choir participant[3]).

When Florence was no longer able to attend the choir sessions, she and Fred came to see me together, for more personalised weekly music therapy sessions at the Raukatauri Music Therapy Centre[4]. Here we sang, played instruments and reminisced together each Tuesday afternoon.

Today I sang and strummed 'Kumbaya', a link with the choir repertoire, and again it was a joy to hear Florence's harmonies. Rather than a set sequence of verses, I sang lyrics that described us. 'Here we are … someone's singing, smiling, sleepy.' Florence enjoyed the whole song and there was a nice sense of being together.

Fred's suggestion of 'Marching to Pretoria' gave me some homework as the song was new to me. Today our voices, melody, rhythm, harmony, drums and cymbal brought the words to life. 'I'm with you and you're with me, and so we will march together.' And then more quietly we hummed and sang, 'Peace is flowing like a river … love is flowing … joy is flowing …'

Florence continues to play the piano by ear in music therapy and at home. Today she again played that decisive right hand melody, with left hand bass and chords, a song familiar to Fred, but we could not identify it. Florence repeated from the beginning several times, seeming a little frustrated that she couldn't quite remember the ending. I joined in, playing the melody on the violin while Florence again played this song on the piano. She then accepted a turn on the violin and played long notes on the A and D strings.

When playing became gradually harder for Florence, Fred handed on the family piano to their son David. However, awareness and perception continue long after people are able to perform or verbally describe complex music. Our focus shifted to Florence's continued interest in singing and rhythm. Other instruments also offered new experiences – guitar, drums, cymbal, tambourine, windchimes, tuned percussion – and improvisation (spontaneous play) offered a form of self-expression that did not depend on memory or verbal communication.

We are sharing the guitar, Florence strumming while I finger the chords. Fred too takes a turn, holding the guitar conventionally, then also flat, exploring open strings and fingering new pitches. Over this Florence and I add some drumbeats. Florence taps around the edge of her drum, counting the beats. She expresses interest and surprise, 'Oh!' when I play more rhythmically. Fred has also become an active musician, enjoying novel instruments such as windchimes, autoharp and ethnic percussion instruments. Florence enjoys his curiosity, but has another kind of 'Oh!' when his drum and cymbal playing is a little loud for her taste!

I set out the tuned percussion; the wooden xylophone, the resonant metallophone and the brighter glockenspiel. I remove the B and F bars to create a pentatonic scale. This avoids discordant sounds and the spaces sometimes suggest melodic patterns. Florence taps out 'Mary had a little lamb', looking satisfied at playing the complete song. When I continue to play a steady pulse and melodic phrases, Florence becomes bolder, more creative, exploring contrasting high and low sounds. The multisensory qualities of the instruments seem important too, not only sounding but also touching and feeling the rough surface of the tambourine and the polished wooden xylophone bars. I turn to the piano, matching Florence's tempo and enriching the improvisation with rhythm, tonal colours, melody and harmony. I sometimes hum and sing. This flexible meandering between a clear

musical structure and a more fluid stream of musical consciousness,
is characteristic of improvisational music therapy. I switch from a
march rhythm to a lilting three, and Florence's continuing perception
of metre and rhythm prompts her to comment 'Now a waltz!'

Occasionally, as during the earlier choir sessions, we invited visiting family members to join us in the music therapy room. Fred's sister came, and joined us in singing, playing and enjoying time together. Two grandchildren visiting from overseas participated in some sessions, a relaxed way to spend time together with an enjoyable, undemanding musical focus. Their initial hesitancy about limited musical skills was quickly allayed, as music therapy does not require participants to have any prior musical experience.

After a period of singing and playing we chat and Fred reminisces about
times past. Florence listens, nodding encouragement and prompting
him: 'You say it!' Fred's stories bring Florence much pleasure, whether
or not she understands every word or remembers every detail. We
hear from Fred about Florence's fondness for her grandfather, her love
of children and roses, their move to New Zealand and their pride in
their children and grandchildren.

Eventually it became more difficult for Florence to get in and out of the car and it seemed that our work would end. However, we were able to arrange for music therapy at home. We sat in the lounge, enjoying beautiful sea views and singing in harmony, as Fred relaxed next to us. This would turn out to be our final time together.

Throughout our lives we create memories for others. Our music, particularly songs, helped Florence to remember moments in her life, to experience and express peace, love and joy through songs and shared moments. I am glad that Fred asked me to record some sessions and make a DVD of video clips to share with their family. I, in turn, remember Florence's smile lighting up the room, her joyful singing, and moments of connection and humour when Florence, Fred and I sang and played together.

Notes

1. My memories of Florence are illustrated by adapted excerpts from my music therapy notes, presented in italics.

2. www.cbr.auckland.ac.nz/choir

3. Quotations from choir participants are drawn from the University of Auckland's SPICCATO research: Talmage, A., Ludlam, S., Leão, S., Fogg-Rogers, L., & Purdy, S.C. (2013). Leading the CeleBRation Choir: The Choral Singing Therapy protocol and the role of the music therapist in a social singing group for adults with neurological conditions. *New Zealand Journal of Music Therapy* 12, 7-50.

4. www.rmtc.org.nz

Choral Singing Therapy for People Living with Neurological Conditions:

The CeleBRation Choir at the University of Auckland's Centre for Brain Research

Alison Talmage, Shari Storie and Roger Hicks

Singers gather on Monday afternoons at the University of Auckland, Tamaki Campus. The Centre for Brain Research (CBR) is the place to be, and choral singing is therapy for this social singing group of people living with neurological conditions and their supporters. Led by registered music therapists Alison Talmage and Shari Storie, members from across Auckland join the CeleBRation Choir for many different reasons, and singing together is foremost. With a love of rock and jazz, Roger Hicks joined the choir to improve his strength of voice, tone and breathing, and hoped to slow any decline associated with his Parkinson's through singing. Roger, Alison and Shari were inspired by the choir's SPICCATO Research Outcomes Song (lyrics by Alison, see below), written to disseminate findings of interviews with choir members, to share more about singing and their experiences of what Monday afternoons at the CBR are all about.

Don't sing

Roger Hicks[1]

Don't sing said the teacher don't sing
The little boy stood alone in the crowd surrounded by friends who stood
    all around
He wanted to sing, he liked all the songs
And with his friends was singing along

You can't hold a note
Chalk on blackboard
Gravel on glass
You're just not musical
This isn't for you

'Lip-synch the words' that's what she said. Its all in your head but don't
    make a sound
Don't sing said the teacher don't sing

As he grew older
At parties, family gatherings and things
There were the songs that everyone sings
Happy Birthday and God save the Queen
But the boy knew his place in the scheme of things
Don't sing said the boy I don't sing

I'm getting old, the body shows age
The brain, once so quick, is now on low power
Words are there on the tip of my tongue
They don't come easy like when I was young

My voice is gruff, croaky and quiet
The voice is so faint I cannot be heard
Frustrating, lonely and oh so absurd

I've asked all the people who ought to know
The doctors, researchers and scientists, therapists and psychologists too
Tell me please What can I do

Sing, they all said, just sing

So I sang and my breathing and voice are better
When I sing my words can often be heard
And I am part of the crowd, not alone, as we all share the pleasure of
    musical words

Through these kids by my side I look through the time telescopic and see
    the boy in the past as a dream

Sing I said to myself just sing

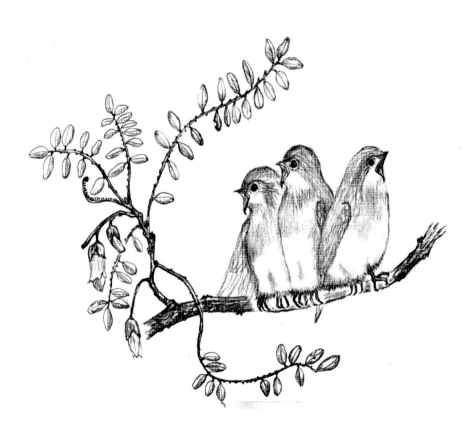

The sounds of a choir CeleBRated

Shari Storie

in the *C*ar I sing - readying, refining, steadying my breathing.
a spoken hum *E*merges as my heels echo across the campus lobby, many are there already.
some cheeky *L*aughter as a finger taps on a watch, warm surrounding tones of greeting,
an *E*xigent voice or two capture me as I clang my music stand loose,
a reassuring *B*urst of tinkled ivories as a volunteer sets up the digital piano,
gentle natter *R*efocused as the projector screen unrolls and I gauge the room -
to instigate *A*nimated, activating strums of a G-chord, or gradually welcome, settle?
are voices *T*hin, stretched and flat or fruity, robust and full of steady breath? I listen,
haere mai, in *I*ndigenous tongue the session has begun. Forty brought together to sing yet
increasingly *O*pen to being operatic gorillas with tiger faces and buzzy-bee tongues zealously
engaged; '*N*o!' sometimes resounding against tongue twister or sung numbered sequence

yet *C*hallenge sought, eager agreement toward two-part well-known round,
the rustle of *H*igh arms or tapped knees for every word of *My Bonnie* starting with B.
proud *O*wnership as they announce their choice of song, familiarity and preference
heard *I*n the strength of their voices – alongside pace, pitch, arrangement and repetition.
identity *R*epresented in resolute defence of original lyrics, artists' rhythms debated,

meaning and *S*ignificance expressed - both sung and shared afterwards, respect, dignity held.
discussions *I*n the refreshment break reverberate with friendship, care and welcome for
visitors, *N*ew members and those six-years-confident. 'Sh, sh' bantered to refocus some,
the *G*roup returns to sing. One's singing is faltering, our eyes meet, my lips model;
volume fades, *I* adapt and revise key and tempo and the volume rises; group rhythm out of sync,
chaining *N*oticeably entrains voices with guitar. *Now is the Hour* brings reflection and farewell, we
celeBRate the *G*ains, the sounds of wellbeing, mood, quality of life, breathing, voice and people.

Choir diary

Alison Talmage

12.45 - driving,
Crawling along the motorway,
Humming today's songs;
Travel and mobility barriers on my mind.

1.25 - arriving,
Parking in a far corner, rushing to be on time,
Guitar in hand;
Slowing my pace to walk alongside.

1.30 – preparing,
Volunteers are already setting up
Chairs, piano, name badges, afternoon tea;
Collaborating - or how would we manage?

1.45 - greeting
Old and new friends in song,
Melody and harmony, humming and lyrics,
Haere mai!

1.50 – warming up
Our bodies and voices,
Noticing our breathing, posture, mood;
Exploring new songs, sounds, harmonies.

2.25 – chatting
Over afternoon tea,
Friendship and fellowship,
Voices and more.

2.40 – *Why are we waiting?*
They tap their watches,
Raise their voices,
Raise eyebrows and smiles.

2.45 – Requesting
Old favourites or something new.
'That one again!'
'Oh, not again!'
Negotiating,
Encouraging, finding courage.

3.15 – Ending,
Now is the hour,
Shalom,
Goodnight Irene,
We'll meet again
Next week.

Choir is

Alison Talmage

Choir is all of us in a song.
A song is stories, memories, emotions.
Emotions are my ups and downs, a melody.
Melody is sounds in space and time.
Time is patience, pacing, practice.
Practice is never giving up.
Giving up is not an option.
Options are having a choice, a voice.
Voice is advocacy, not being silenced.
Silence is anticipation, reflection, frustration.
Frustration is words on the tip of my tongue.
Tongue, teeth, lips should make consonants.
Consonants are la-la-la and doo-be-doo-be-doo.
Oo is a vowel, a-e-i-o-u, A-E-I-O-U.
You raise me up, you'll never walk alone, you are my sunshine.
Sunshine is light, warmth, hope.
Hope is friendship and fellowship, my place in the choir.

My brain

Roger Hicks[1]

With apologies to Adrian Mitchell

I wandered in the CBR[2] and handed them my brain
Can you overhaul, 'cos its playing up again?
They prodded it and poked it and threw it on the floor
Its well past its use-by date, its broke and that's for sure
We can't trade in on a new one 'cos this model's obsolete
The power supply is wrong and the valves are incomplete
We'll add it to the brain bank and put it on display
The sign will read 'one old brain, that's really had its day'

It is **my** brain,
           not a frog or a dog,
                     and I want it back again

You and I were happy once, not so many years ago
But we were torn apart because my brain was going slow
I really don't know what I'll do, the future's not that clear
A life alone without you is something that I fear
So tell me that you love me and hold me in your arms
We can face the world as one, when shielded by your charms
I took my brain for granted, it wasn't very fair
And now the damn thing's broken and lost beyond repair

It is **my** brain,
           not a frog or a dog,
                     and I want it back again

Think

Roger Hicks[1]

Cogito ergo Sum
I think therefore I am
… At least I think I am!

Here inside my head I am who I think I am,
I am the reality of my own thinking,
Reality is what I am.

My world is what I think about,
I am irreplaceably part of my world, part of who I am.

They say part of my brain is dying.
Is my reality different?
Am I thinking less?
It is getting more difficult to think,
Does this mean I am less?

Cogito ergo Sum
I think therefore I am
Sum ergo cogito
I am therefore I think
I think about
            Green fields and beech woods on summer days
            Snow drifts in country lanes
            Children playing in sand and surf
I think about the future

Cogito ergo Sum
Sum ergo canto
I think therefore I am
I am therefore I sing
… at least I think I can sing

Lost in song is my changing reality as my brain thinks less and I am
   less.

I am music and song. Canto ergo sum. I sing therefore I am.
I am inside my head where music has trod new pathways.
Why and How?
I don't think, I just enjoy the effects of music
 … I just am

SPICCATO[3] research outcomes song

Alison Talmage[4]

Tune: On my way to Canaan Land (Trad.)

Monday afternoons at university,
The CBR is the place to be,
Choral singing is our therapy,
    Oh, we all love the CeleBRation Choir!

SPICCATO is our research name,
Questionnaires and tests, and more of the same,
It's bringing us international fame,
    Oh, we all love the CeleBRation Choir!

Our study showed people will take part,
And test their voices at the start,
In the middle of term and before they depart,
    Oh, we all love the CeleBRation Choir!

Group data show, by a stroke of luck,
You can sing in the choir and you won't feel stuck,
Your words will feel simpler to construct
    Oh, we all love the CeleBRation Choir!

Your voice will be LOUDER, tuneful and strong,
When you've lots to say, your breath will be long____,
You know you've a voice, and you are not wrong,
    Oh, we all love the CeleBRation Choir!

Songs from your culture help you sing along,
Though travelling far makes it harder for some,
If you have a carer who is ready to come,
 Oh, you will love the CeleBRation Choir!

Quality of life is better if you sing,
Surrounded by friends and all the love they bring,
Singing cheers you up, it's a positive thing,
 Oh, we all love the CeleBRation Choir!
 Yes, we all love the CeleBRation Choir!

~

Notes

1. Poems by Roger Hicks. Copyright © 2016 by Roger Hicks. Printed with permission from Roger Hicks.

2. Centre for Brain Research

3. SPICCATO is the acronym of a 2010-2011 study at the Centre for Brain Research – Stroke and Parkinson's: Community Choirs and Therapeutic Outcomes.

4. Copyright © 2011 by University of Auckland Centre for Brain Research. Previously published in the New Zealand Journal of Music Therapy (2013). Reprinted with permission of the University of Auckland and Music Therapy New Zealand.

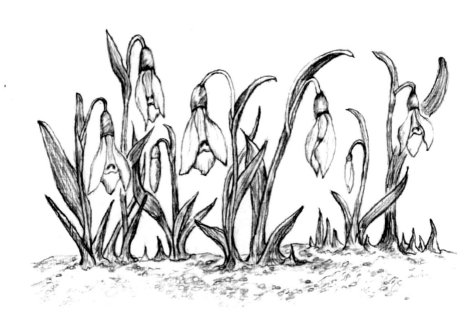

III
Personal Journeys

Polyphony
Shari Storie

Blonde ponytail stands
In a local whare
Swings a ball of newspaper wrapped
in plastic bag, tied with tawny wool.
Looks, scared by pāua eyes on the walls
Worries, eating food from the ground not understood.
Sings with the large, loud men and women as they stomp,
Unsure, but starting to ease

Blonde ponytail sits
In a classroom
Hears Treaty - Mentality of savages, of
Bringing civilisation, technology,
Trade, advantages, new promises;
Reality of pests, mistreatment, disrespect,
Fighting, disease, death – translation lost.
There, but heard it before

Blonde ponytail meets
In a university seminar
Shares family history
Of pākehā dairy farm reclaimed, unfair;
Met with distaste, offence, discord,
Questions why her cultural heritage
Isn't heard, respected.
Disconnected, but acknowledges dissonance

Blonde ponytail watches
In a music therapy room
Surprised, intrigued by the young
Pākehā – enthusiastic, determined, at ease,
Sings, knowing all of the words of *Poi E*
Stomps, inviting, encouraging, inspiring
Others to join in. Separate, politely
Accompanying, but challenged

Blonde bob begins to learn
In a room of fellow questioners
Playing 'the Māori strum'
Questions why recent immigrants
Know more, sing more, care more, consider more
Than the Kiwi girl who grew up here
Wonders why we can't just all be Kiwis.
Irresolute, but at the door

Blonde bob begins to reflect
In a supervisory space
Absorbs that heritage and multi-cultural experience
Shape and influence response.
Knows her mihi will always be of Mount Egmont
That holds her grandparents - but
Pronounces Tah-rah-nah-kee with a rolling 'r'.
Edging, but takes a step

Blonde bob begins to listen
In the waiting area, the lounge, the room
Surrounded by others in need, now
Meaning holds importance beyond therapeutic spaces
The underlying, the overarching, behaviour, actions, words
Holistically valued, held meaningful
How could one hear and yet not listen?
Present, but still seeking

Blonde bob begins to feel
In the present world
Had heard the story, could tell the story,
But does one feel the story of the case moth?
Does the pūtōrino invite, allow the player?
Her metal flute, bought when young, warm;
A kōauau made, sound not yet evoked.
Lost, but inviting translation

Blonde bun leads
Waiata, swings poi, no longer worried except
In the future land of the long white cloud;
When will the taonga pūoro emerge
From its forgotten cocoon in sound?
Surprise, acceptance, discord all valid.
One Kiwi forages, seeks,
Moved and emerging

From Singer-Songwriter to Music Therapist
Ajay Castelino

Where it began

The room was dark and smoky with a wooden stage at the far end. I approached the bar, acoustic guitar in hand, and put my name on the list for a spot under the lights. After two hours of listening to other wannabe musicians, it was my turn on stage. Nervously I settled in and worked my way through the three songs I'd prepared. The audience, punters just like me, worked their Dolly Parton nine to five jobs and then crawled in here for a stab at their secret desires and aspirations. Mine was the lure of the creative muse, the song-writing type. Every morning I would push it away and engineer door lock designs at a desk that paid the rent. But as the sun said goodnight, Mr Muse would unlock a secret door and tempt me with yet another title or witty line, urging me to delve deeper into the whirlpool of rhymes and story-telling. The expression, the emotion and the drug of letting my heart out in front of strangers was a craving that was hard to resist.

Chasing a bigger high, I gambled on longer sets, competitions and elusive record deals. Some of these did cross my path. But up ahead on this windy road I also saw lots of late nights, lots of 'who knows who the most' and lots of image make-overs. The thirst for just writing and performing was overcast by shadows of a machine bigger than myself.

Drudging back to the road most travelled, I meekly got on with day-jobbing and the general busyness of flatting with a bunch of mates. One cold winter's evening, seven years into this round-about of stages and songs, I was busy cooking dinner. Suddenly, there was a strange word blaring from the TV, *Music Therapy*. Rushing out to the lounge I heard the six o'clock news reporter talking about a new music therapy centre starting in Auckland. How interesting! Jumping onto the computer I searched for this word. Hmm, this thing seemed to involve music, which I enjoyed, and psychology, which I enjoyed. It seemed to be a nine to five job which would mean no more smoky pubs and late nights. It also used music to help people rather than sell beers. This was beginning to look good. And there was a training course right here in Wellington!

Booking an appointment I ran along to meet the head of the course. So, I'm asked: 'Have you got a Bachelors or Licentiate in music?' Hmm … no. 'Have you got a Bachelors in Psychology or relevant experience?' Hmm … no. 'Okay, then', I was told, 'get them and come back and we can talk.' Yikes! I like the sound of this music therapy thing but how will I get all this stuff?

Ideas started to whirl around my head. There were two requirements, the music qualifications thing and the psychology qualifications thing. I had already done a few psychology papers but did I want to do a whole degree in it? I was not so keen. But this music thing, well I could use this as an excuse to study music and work in the field full-time so that I can get into the course. Now, that sounds like a good plan!

The long and winding road

And so I left my day job, packed my bags, got a working holiday visa and moved to London to become a professional musician, thinking: 'It's best to start anew in a city where no-one knows my name.' Transitioning from a hobbyist to a full-time musician was a shock to the system! I was always patted on my back for my guitar playing skills, but now, compared to the professionals I was auditioning with, I felt like a cheap knock-off guitar in a Gibson showroom. I quickly understood that getting a guitar solo note perfect was no longer the aim, getting it good enough for the punters and learned before tonight's gig was what mattered. Starting to do grades on guitar was a revelation as Grade Four suddenly felt like an impossible task and I had to get to a licentiate level in three years!

In a bid to get music therapy related experience, I tried becoming a teaching assistant. Eventually I got some contract work though an agency. Coming from the corporate world, I wore a suit to my first day at work with a 10-year-old child with autism. The agency called later that evening and said the school staff found me a little distant from the child and would prefer me not to return. That was a good start! This was a new planet with very different outlooks from the corporate world. Luckily lessons were learned and I wore more appropriate clothing to the next contract where I ended up staying for three months. Using this experience, I eventually managed to get a job as a music teacher in a school for children with special needs.

A short vignette: What do I do?

Part of my teaching duties involved individual music lessons. It was while working with Jack, a 10-year-old boy with attention deficit hyperactivity disorder (ADHD), that I first wondered if I could use a music therapy approach to help his learning. Entering the music room, he would flit from one instrument to another, never staying anywhere for longer than two minutes. Teaching concepts like keeping a beat were challenging for him to grasp. I wondered if music therapy may be a more appropriate medium for Jack. Music therapy should be able to help him learn ways to extend his attention span, which seemed like a prerequisite to engage in more learning based music activities. I finally had an opportunity to try out my wannabe personality of 'Music Therapist!' And then I stopped. I had absolutely no idea what to do! So here I sat, ready to engage, but with no idea where to start.

During these years, I didn't have much time for song writing. It was more a time of learning the craft of music making and how to work in settings where music therapists are likely to trade their wares. It felt right to set aside a singer-songwriter focus for now. There was a lot to learn in each of these two seemingly disparate fields of music and therapy that I hoped to eventually marry together in the profession of music therapy.

I do need some education

After three years and 12-hour days of studying and working in London town, I knocked on Wellington's door again and this time they let me in! For the next two years I studied the use of music as a therapy. While on placement at a school for students with special needs, I was engaging in music making with my client while being observed by my supervisor.

After the session, my supervisor asked me to describe my aim for the session. I was unsure; I had assumed that engaging in music with this child would automatically assist them. I began to understand the role of assessment, planning and delivery of sessions. This revelation, along with many others, helped me piece together the parts of the puzzle and understand how to proceed in situations similar to the one described above with Jack.

It was good to have my experiences as a musician before starting my training. Training to be a music therapist is a full-time job and having my musician part of my music therapist skills sorted out meant that I could focus primarily on learning how to use these skills in a therapeutic context. I also began to song-write again, but from a different perspective. Rather than writing for myself, I was now writing to meet the needs of others. It was reinvigorating to use music with such a purposeful focus.

Who are you?

Two years later I had a piece of paper to prove I was an official music therapist! Ever since that day, there is a question I have been asked and will continue to be asked for the rest of my professional life, 'Music therapist! Wow, hmm … so what exactly do you do?' 'Well, I am still trying to figure out the answer myself! Music therapy work lies within psychological realms and therefore concrete and absolute is relative to where, when and with whom. To help me ground myself I initially tried approaching it from the perspective of a medical drug. Teach me the dosage of scales and chords to cure a broken heart. I soon learned that music, like people, is esoteric. The possibilities are endless. Each patient has a unique mind and with it, his or her own set of musical associations and reactions. One person's song of joy was another's song of sorrow.

A short vignette: Song sung blue

A few years into my practice, I was carrying out a music therapy group session at a rest home for older people. I sang my greeting song and then proceeded with the session. After about 15 minutes, an elderly gentlemen said, with a lilt in his voice: 'Play me *Danny Boy*, music man.' He told me it reminded him of happy childhood days back home in Ireland. As I sang, I noticed the cheery smile on his face. As I observed the other people in the group, I noticed a lady with a single tear in her eye. After the song, I turned to the lady and commented that she seemed sad. 'The song reminds me of my dear husband, young man. He is now no longer with me.' She replied through a stream of tears. After the session I approached her and offered the opportunity for some individual work to help her work through her grief. Accepting this offer, we proceeded to a quiet room and improvised on instruments to help express feelings that she found difficult to verbalise. She gently tapped the xylophone and shed a few quiet tears while I supported her musical expression on a hand drum. I often don't need words in a session, music does the talking for me.

Feelin' groovy

The above vignette taught me that music therapy had to be person-centred. Being a music therapist was different from being a musician or performer. As a musician I was more centred on my musical preferences but as a music therapist my focus was on the needs of the clients. The commonplace terminology 'tuning in' took on a whole new meaning in music therapy. Initially I found myself in an incongruent place to my clients and had to work hard on learning how to tune in to what they were feeling and present appropriate musical experiences. As a musician, this was an exciting revelation. The experience of 'tuning in' and 'locking in' to the groove of a band was transformed as I explored locking into the groove of a person, using this as a basis for our joint exploration within music. In a band, locking into the groove is what gives the performance its X-Factor, it is what separates great bands from background music. I now realised that before therapy can happen, the groove must first be realised.

When I meet new clients, especially cognitively able clients, most cautiously enter the music therapy room and listen, in an off-handed way to the music I play. They listen to the technical level of my playing or my ability to play their song requests. Then slowly, the sun begins to shine and it feels a lot warmer in the room. They open up and begin to engage in musical conversations and improvisations. The music comes first and the therapy follows. I feel that having a solid musician background is key to forming that initial bond with my clients which allows for the trust that can lead into therapy. I then work within psychological realms and use my musical knowledge to facilitate the use of music as an alternative to a talking therapy to enable expression and release for the client.

Found what I'm looking for

A part of my professional life that took some getting used to was dealing with the unknown. I had goals on which I was working with the client, however, tuning into the client's current presentation could mean a very different session than anticipated! This sense of the unknown was scary but also exciting. It was a pivotal difference for me between taking on a music teaching profession and music therapy. I felt that in music therapy I was getting a greater opportunity to flex my improvisation muscles.

A huge part of this journey has been deciphering what made music therapy different from other therapies. I often felt that other therapies were much easier to explain. Physiotherapy was about the body, speech and language therapy was about … speech and language. But was music therapy about music? I discovered, not really. However, herein lies the beauty of this profession. I discovered that the niche of music therapy rests in the crevice where talking therapies were less effective. These were settings where the clients were not able to speak either due to cognitive or physical impairment, or where self-expression was easier through nonverbal means without the challenge of finding the words. Within this space, I learned about the beauty of music as a language. It was a language that could traverse traditional speech to relate directly at the core of the being. Musically, it felt like the truest use of music. Even for verbal clients, music therapy offered a space to express feelings, sometimes hidden. The art of song writing allowed me to facilitate thoughts and expressions into song. My studio skills allowed me to assist clients to record these expressions and have a personal record of the experience they wished to share. I also got the opportunity to write songs with specific goals in mind. Rather than just self-expression, it was song writing used to deliver specific goals. This has spilled over into me recording and sharing these song findings via releasing music therapy song albums. So, here I am now, a registered music therapist, using my passion for music to help people and provide myself with a much richer and deeper experience and a reason to continue to play and write.

Manawarū ana au

Nolan Hodgson

My blue eyes sweaty in that ripe silage stench
Hot scones folding into sweaty chequered shirts
Into lanolin laced bales and stale sheep droppings
From woolshed to bike shed to cowshed to a watershed

My blue eyes spying out between the branches
From tree hut to swimming pool
Stashed plastic bottles for when we need to *pop a Mangere*
Following barberry hedges up into the bush
And revolving beneath a tawa canopy
On a yellow ropeswing with a rātā vine seat

My blue eyes driving daily past Orākau
Knowing nothing of 'Rewi's last stand'
And the corrupted histories we inhabit
Learning that books forget as easily as we remember
And things are best kept in song

My blue eyes swapping silent 'kia ora'
With a fluent three-year-old
Locking with kaumātua before hongi
Allowing my self to be drawn in

My blue eyes inhaling oral histories
Discovering PAPA-TU-A-NUKU with Hone Tuwhare
And rewriting her in chalk beneath my bare feet
To get her off the page and onto some concrete in the city

My blue eyes comparing an ancestor's whare in Poland
With a grainy photo taken by my grandfather
A thatched roof stretching for the floor
Poached cabbage parcels for dinner
And coal dust hanging lazily in the twilight

My blue eyes adjusting to the light
In a wharenui far removed from my experience
But still familiar and filling slowly with a reo
That I only missed by two generations

My blue eyes devouring kaimoana as it's laid out
Savouring the watercress still in bed underwater
Relishing a butter laden loaf soaking in gravy
Searching for the way inside a kina

My blue eyes avoiding their gaze
So I don't have to stand up and speak
Hiding behind my inexperience, my pākehātanga
But knowing I will be bound to use it

My blue eyes practising pūkana in the mirror
Closing to internally rehearse
Those taonga that I need for more
Than entertainment

My blue eyes tracing my musical whakapapa
From a piano accordion in Te Urewera
To the church organ at Manawarū
Anxious, enraptured, ecstatic, uneasy

My blue eyes resolute as my voice emerges
Shaky and mistake laden
But singing because it's necessary
With an ever increasing repertoire
Of places and situations that depend upon song

My blue eyes sharing and attempting
To remain open and inviting
Present and aware during
My work

My blue eyes giving over
To my ears, to any other sensations
That let me gain acquaintance with
Whatever my blue eyes cannot see

Six of the Many Understandings that Music Therapy Journeys gave me

Carolyn Ayson

1. It starts with the hope that we can find each other in the music

If arpeggios were the leaps you're proud to have made
If ostinatos were the habits you wish you could break
If staccatos were the people who left you too soon
If chromatic runs were the creeping fears that chase you
If demi semi quavers ran your thoughtful 4 am awakenings
If 4/4 was made from the daily routines you march on
If crescendos were the mountains you rolled sideways down
If slurs were the umbrellas that met your sun and rain
If rests were the moments that took your breath away, hand over mouth
If counterpoint was the Lego City you made with another
If rhythm was the manner in which you held it all together
If motifs were your ancestors reminding you of family threads
If bar lines were the wide door frames for your voice to sneak out
If tied notes were your eyes working together to focus on a dream
If minims were the spaces in your heart not blackened

By hearing a piece of your music, I could trace your outline for
        the first time
Then you could show me how to colour it in,
                        with the symphonies to come.

2. Fun is seriously important

Fun:
adj. Amusing, entertaining, enjoyable.
The onlooking allied health professional said one thing only:
'That looked like fun.'
The antonym of which is 'serious'.

Serious:
adj. Characterised by careful consideration or application.
Were my sessions with Rose taken as seriously as I thought they should be?

--

I remember how Rose graduated from sitting on her mumma's knee,
to sitting by herself on the cushion.
She stopped running.
She sat still.

I remember 'Old McDonald' and the first time her lips formed a circle
at just the right time:
I sang, 'E I E I',
and she sang, 'O'.

I remember the choices Rose made when she realised
each object represented a different song:
She put the frog hat on.
I sang 'Galoop'.

I remember her excitement when through the kazoo the wind blowing sound
turned into a merry tune:
She learned that instead of blowing,
you could sing through.

There were new movements learned.
Bowing violins tremolo, squeezing accordions terrifically.
There were new words understood:
Up, down, stop, wait, drum.

The sessions were more than just fun.

But then I remembered the trampoline positioned music summer jams,
Sun shiny faces.
The bird-cheering fans.

I remembered the fluffy Incy Wincy spider puppet.
Crawling past her turned up lip.
Crawling past mine.

I remembered her favourite book that was set to song.
Rose turning the pages.
Me singing along.

I remembered her excited squeals when sighting the violin case.
The sound of Christmas.
Every week she'd celebrate.

There were jack-in-the-box surprises.
Parachute gliding up, down - one of us hiding.
Silly synthesiser sounds rising.
Both of us smiling.

This fun that we shared was the thread that kept us knitting another knot.
It was the enthusiasm that slapped Rose's hand hard against her chest
signing for more.
And if it were not, we would fall flat.
For fun is baking soda to the human spirit.
It needed to be, not an optional extra, a necessity.
And I know this because I stared at Rose's petals, as she showed me what made
them open up.

My question shouldn't be, were our sessions taken seriously, but was fun taken
seriously enough?

Our sessions were more than just developmental goals,
they were SERIOUSLY FUN.

3. What's important is not always measurable

Together you danced to my guitar.
You and your mum,
moving as one you were held in love's arms.
Your blond Goldilocks hair, with blue eyes to match,
made a picture so perfect.

Sometimes you would sleep.
Exhausted after the earthquakes of seizures, you were still.
Over the smell of peppermint tea, your mum and I talked.
Waiting … hoping … that you would wake
and together gently dance to my guitar.

Snaked behind your ear a nasal gastric tube rests,
reminding us of the trouble within.
I held the vomit bucket many times, too many times for a child so small,
And then, after the warmth of a face cloth,
together you danced to my guitar.

Tuesdays were a busy day.
Conductive education, then acupuncture, then me.
I would sing hi,
while your mum ate with speed,
so that together you could dance to my guitar.

We did other things too.
You learnt to grasp a shaker and make the chimes move.
The sounds in the room created by you.
Exercises matched carefully with music and songs.
But you beamed most of all, when together you danced to my guitar.

I struggled, I did, to write your reports.
So much so that I stopped.
Progress had little place here, every week was played by ear.
I could feel the importance of the sessions, but on paper only one thing felt
pleasing to write.
That together you danced to my guitar.

At five years old, you passed away.
No longer here, but your message remains.
'We thought we were here for Ella, but Ella was here for us,'
your mum explained.
She was right, you taught me so much,
when together you danced to my guitar.

In amongst all of your struggles, there were moments of smiles to be had.
You did not need to reach any particular milestone or be better or more able.
For meaningful moments were there and shared within the hour.
Some of the happiest memories your mum will cherish, she said, were made
from the singing and movements.
Illuminating that which was most important

That together you danced.

4. I won't always know, and I often don't

You sat behind the drums.
Cymbal throwing gold light on your nine-year-old face, and you asked:
'Do all the people that do music with you have problems?'
An innocent question with a weight so important, that I struggled to hold it enough to answer.

- I wanted to say, 'No, they don't have problems, they have special gifts and abilities that we are finding in our music.'
- I wanted to say, 'No, they wear capes sewn from their point of difference that make them fly in a way like no other.'

Then I thought this might make you feel alone in the struggles you told me you had. So,

- I wanted to say, 'Yes, we all have problems that we need help with at times to fix.'
- I wanted to say, 'Yes, music meets their cuts, like ointment, to heal their problems.'

Then I thought this might make you feel bad about yourself if your problem leaves a permanent mark. So,

- I wanted to say, 'No, they don't have problems, society has problems in accommodating difference.'
- I wanted to say, 'The square peg being squeezed into a round hole is not the problem, the shape of the hole is.'

Then I thought this might make you feel powerless, that you have no control or agency in what bothers you so. So,

- I wanted to say, 'Well, yes and no. They don't have problems but they might think they do which makes the monster come to life.'
- I wanted to say, 'In music we find ways to turn the made up scary monster story into a new fluffy cuddly one. Like what the musical 'Wicked' does for the Wicked Witch of the West'.

But to tell you all of those answers would make you as confused as I.
So instead of determining whether it is you, I, or we that have a problem,
Or whether a problem exists or was created like Santa,
My silence told you everything:
That I'm still working it all out.

5. Taking care of your self is important for others

Dear new graduate self,

After the graduation celebration with Champagne in your hand,
karaoke killing the melodies of songs with laughing larrikins.
You will wake up officially a therapist.

Rubbing your eyes to focus on the opportunities before you,
in equal measure will sit nerves and excitement
in the pit of your padded stomach.

Session plans read and re-read: a security blanket for the mind,
will only later be discovered as inadequate.
Free falling as you see what else you missed.

Naturally, you start to spend more time in the professional persona.
Talking the talk, walking the walk.
Trying to be, blemish free.

Gathering success like trinkets of reassurance.
Conference papers written, committees sat on, full time work load
happening.
It will all be happening!

As you fill these shoes, more of your sense of worth attaches to that
professional self.
Accomplishments add to your sticker chart.
Showing this is where you are.

Society's mantra of more is more, less is less, is hard to resist.
As your report writing steals another lie in Sunday with your love
'cause it seems you can never do enough.

Enough.
Go gently.
While remembering,
You are as human as your clients and as worthy of your time.
In the ticking when you clock out.
Stop.

The space has something to offer:
A finger to your pulse reminder that human is the only way to work.
For strangling it would be like a rabbit trying to gallop with a horse.

See your flaws,
Your cracks position the client as an equal,
Pulling you down the ladder of expert to sit on the floor with another.

Feel your hurt,
So you can practice kindness to yourself first.
For then the spilled blood of another will be met with the gentleness you
had when you bled.

Stand in your uncertainty,
With supervision enhancing the flexibility that comes with feet stumbling.
You will then value these meetings as necessary groceries to feed
the mobile mind.

Sit and watch,
Still yourself by watching a snail eat, a spider spin.
Growing patience and appreciation within the small moments jet-setters
miss in therapeutic travels.

Be a comedian,
Pause to rattle ribs with laughter for lightness.
To create helium filled lungs to rise from the depths of challenging topics
that challenge clients.

Touch reached out hands,
They knit a prosperous parachute to cushion your fall.
Grasping that 'people who need people are the luckiest people' squashes
client pitying.

Taste your worth,
From the cocktails of cuddles, shared jokes, and sanded toes.
For then in the moments of work related woes, or cessation, your
self-esteem won't cycle the sink.

Rest when weary,
Don't ignore the heaviness of holding up your body.
Ingrained pacing fiddles the faucets to get sessions more
functionally flowing.

Do fun,
Pottery, poetry, paragliding, whatever starts sparks igniting.
Awaking the role of playfulness to start others' engines doing wheelies off in
new directions.

Take time out as part of your PD[1],
So there is the time to *see, feel, stand, sit, be, touch, taste, rest* and *do* you.
Doing more with less,
The small become the big.

Feel the time the sun gifts.

Then, you will remember what it is to live as you journey
with the life of another.

6. Endings can be therapeutic challenges

'Put your faith in the music'. This mantra, tattooed in training, I contemplate while thinking how this ending may go. Will it be like singing *Auld Lang Syne*? Arms linked dancing cheerfully. Or will it be me holding on too long to make sure you are ready, while *You say goodbye and I say hello, hello, hello*. Will it be like a perfect cadence made from careful calendar countdowns? Or a wave before walking away without looking back over our shoulders? Will it be an interrupted cadence, a sudden loss with goodbyes taken by illness or pulled funding? May we fall on the spiritual Plagal when lost?

For you, none of these endings feel right. Our fingers dance with an origami fortune teller of 'should we' or 'shouldn't we' bring this to a close. Each year that we have spent creating together adds another weight to the thought of ending. Can we no longer imagine what it would be to not see each other in that weekly space? A space that has become a way of life: no longer marked in calendars for it is embedded, not something added.

If we could just feel what the inevitable presence of ending is like, might we stop avoiding it from passing our lips and could you then hear my mumbling attempts? I write about one of my earliest memories of dreading an ending, hoping that my pen will guide me with more insight…

I take off before I know how to land the ride.
Right leg winding back to stroke the concrete, as if hoping to smooth it out.
Skateboard's stomach holding my two-footed meal.
With giddiness I start to go down, trying not to make a meal of it.

From the top of the hill, the street looks long.
Houses stand in rows like spectators as I pass.
Witnessing the journey with their top hats on and different coloured
            personalities.
They encourage me with their constancy.

As time goes on my speed gets faster, and as I go faster time slips away.
I wonder if I can remain balanced during the speed wobbles.
Knees bent, game-face on, I settle in to the whistling wind.
The gushing sound that being in motion makes.

Stones throw a different course to the one I thought.
I lean one way to avoid them, lean another and snap a stick.
Snatch the leaves off a tree to try and plant me somewhere straight,
So the thrill can be grasped.

With reflexes sneezing jumps over cracks and coughing tricks of fun.
All things well, I look up to enjoy the world rush by.
By now I am flying and I wasn't supposed to be.
Only birds can know of this word I'm feeling.

As the path gets shorter, like an old jersey it will wear thin,
Having not as much to offer. Mum calling me in for dinner.
There has always been the knowledge that stopping is inevitable.
But only now do the kneepads and helmet not feel enough.

The rest of my body exposed, I curl up in the nakedness.
Tentatively examining what is to come.
Knowing it is against the nature of things to keep going,
But too scared to try and break in case I fall.

Up until now, wheels carried these legs.
There was not the heavy motionlessness of standing beside the board's edge.
I close my eyes and wish for a slower speed to pull back time,
Because I took off before I knew how to land this ride.

… As my pen stops, I think, is it a bit like this for you? If so, I can offer you my scraped kneepads. They remind me that what felt like a hard end was actually the beginning of new skills and other adventures. Could our end instead be a beginning?

Notes

1. Professional Development (PD)

About the Contributors

Robina Adamson

Robina was formerly a psychopaedic nurse. She studied psychology, New Zealand literature and Māori anthropology at Auckland University. She is qualified in a number of alternative health modalities and has an interest in the study of environmental pollution and its effects on human health, and especially birth defects in children. Robina's beautiful book *The Gift of Mamaku* tells of a powerful and moving spiritual encounter that led to healing for her daughter Mali. In 2016, Robina's poem *The Language of Stones* was arranged for unaccompanied choir by composer Chris Artley especially for New Zealand Choral Federation's '*Sing Aotearoa 2016*'. Robina has lived in the Cook Islands, Fiji and in Western Samoa. Today she lives in Auckland with her daughter and grandchildren and continues to write poetry, draw and illustrate.

Carolyn Ayson

Carolyn Ayson grew up in the town of Timaru, with views of the Southern Alps and summer dips in the Rangitata River. At kindergarten she was prohibited from turning on the stereo, as she would spend her entire playtime dancing and singing along to it. Her teachers encouraged her parents to direct this energy into dance or music lessons. From this grew her love of dancing, playing the piano, singing, and musical theatre. Later in life she learnt to play the violin, guitar and mbira (... or anything that could make a sound). This engagement in music and the performing arts kept her moving through her primary and secondary schooling where she liked to spend more time daydreaming than doing her math sheets. Carolyn went to Victoria University and completed a Bachelor in Music followed by a Master of Music Therapy degree. She had found an enthusiastic focus during these years and obtained a first class masters. Her love of learning continues to grow. She is currently halfway through her PhD. Carolyn has worked with a diverse range of people in her music therapy practice since graduating in 2007. She primarily works with children, their families, and schools. Carolyn enjoys supporting people's passions and interests in sessions and getting to see the unique gifts of each person.

Anne Bailey
Anne has always loved pattern and texture and her artwork is an exploration of these. She has studied botany, zoology and fine arts but it is her love of all things handmade that has led to the creation of her unique mixed media pieces. Each piece is painstakingly hand cut and assembled in fabric and paper. Anne's work draws heavily on her interest in New Zealand's unique fauna and flora and her concerns. You can see more of Anne's work at www.annebailey.co.nz.

Ajay Castelino
Ajay is a New Zealand registered music therapist. He holds a Master of Music Therapy with First Class Honours from Te Kōkī New Zealand School of Music and a Licentiate Teaching Diploma in Electric Guitar from the London College of Music. He has over eight years experience using music therapy in the fields of special needs, mental health and Alzheimer's disease.

Heather Fletcher
Music and theatre have always been my passion. I have sung for as long as I can remember. Learning instruments followed, nurtured by my parents. Then I was introduced to theatre and I had stars in my eyes. This led me to a career in professional theatre. It was while I was doing a multi-sensory hydrotherapy pool show for children with profound and multiple learning difficulties, and a girl with severe cerebral palsy became relaxed enough to walk to the side of the pool following the show, I knew I wanted to train as a music therapist. And so I did - at Bristol University, UK.

A twist of fate then brought me to New Zealand and a career in mental health. I haven't looked back.

Roger Hicks

Roger was born and brought up in Gloucestershire in the West Country of England. He graduated in Mathematics from Bath University and he established his career in the emerging field of electronic computers with technical roles for Rolls Royce jet engines and then with a US computer manufacturer. In the mid-1970s he and his family emigrated to New Zealand to work on one of Muldoon's 'Think Big' projects. The computer industry at this time was still in its infancy in New Zealand. Since then he has held a wide range of roles in the computer, information technology and Internet fields working with government, private industry and academia in technical and management fields. He has been an active participant in the evolution and development of information technology (IT) in the country and internationally. Although now retired IT is still an active interest. Roger was diagnosed with Parkinson's in 2004, and joined the CeleBRation Choir in 2010. He enjoys poetry however this is the first time he has made it available for publication.

Nolan Hodgson

Nolan is a recently qualified music therapist who lives in rural Waikato in the community of Pukeatua. When completing his music therapy qualifications, his Tūhoe and Ngāti Awa whakapapa led him to research the relationship between his music therapy practice and Māori models of health. Initially specialising in working alongside youth in the mental health sector, he now works with people living with dementia. Alongside music therapy, he is also a host at Out in the Styx Guesthouse and spends as much time as possible amongst the native bush and its many inhabitants who cloak Maungatautari, an ecological reserve behind his home.

Libby Johns

After completing a Bachelor of Music, majoring in performance jazz, Libby took two years to travel and dabble with the idea to embark on a new career path. However, curiosity got the better of her and she was drawn back to music to embark on a Master of Music Therapy degree, at Te Kōkī New Zealand School of Music. Libby has worked as a registered music therapist in Auckland, New Zealand, since 2013. Improvisation, playfulness and the 'now' continue to guide Libby's work with children and adults to promote communication and meaningful experiences.

Claire Molyneux

Claire grew up singing songs at the piano with her mother and spent hours recording musical stories into a cassette recorder while her mother taught piano lessons. She moved on to accompanying dance classes and as a rehearsal pianist and musical director for amateur musical theatre. It was not until after training and working for several years as a music therapist that Claire really appreciated the connection between these early experiences and the work she has done for more than 20 years. A deep appreciation of people's stories and experiences, and a desire to work collaboratively guide Claire's work as a music therapist and clinical supervisor.

Shari Storie

On my 20-years of formal music training I draw
Piano, flute, saxophone, voice, guitar, percussion and more
A psychology, statistics and music composition undergrad
The chance to delve into the glorious world of music therapy I then had.

Volunteer assistant to Registered MThs my eyes opened
On to two-years Master's in the windy Wellington with hope and
I was travelling a road diverse with age, strengths, and need,
Response to music, benefit from music, and more indeed!

To schools, a hospital, organisations and homes across Auckland I drive,
Special needs, mental health, neuro-disability and aged care thrive.
Their strengths, goals and their whole person
Central to spaces I think, process and observe in.

With my therapeutic hat on, upon theories I draw -
Psychodynamics, Developmental - to interpret what I heard, saw.
Every person reveals more about how together we can be,
What music can do, how to connect with non-musical need.

And to reflect upon this is a pleasure indeed.

Alison Talmage

Just call me Ali,
Alison Claire Talmage, but
Ali's short, like me.

You ask where I'm from,
England, Wales, Cornwall, NZ,
I call them all home.

I live near the beach,
Walk along the sand, breathing
In, out, the sea air.

I can't imagine
Life without music and song
The sounds and silence,

The thoughts beyond words,
Memories, emotions evoked,
In me, in us all.

Marie Willis

Since the day Marie witnessed an elated audience roused to its feet at the musical climax of a junior wind orchestra performance (within which she played) she knew that her adult work must involve sharing music's power to move people. During her undergraduate Degree in Music she was introduced to the profession of music therapy by her clarinet teacher. A few years later Marie completed a Post Graduate Diploma in music therapy at the Guildhall School of Music and Drama, London, UK. In 2007, Marie flew to the other side of the world to take up a full time position as music therapist at the Raukatauri Music Therapy Centre, Auckland, NZ. In January 2015, Marie took a side-step from working as a therapist, choosing to focus on her other two musical passions; music education and music performance. Marie remains a strong advocate for the profession, and the benefits of music therapy and recognises that her own musical and personal journeys are deeply indebted to those clients and families with whom she shared the power of music.

Glossary

Aotearoa – Māori name for New Zealand
haere mai – welcome, come here
harakeke – flax bush
Hone Tuwhare – New Zealand Māori poet (1922-2008)
hongi – to press noses in greeting, exchange of breath
kaimoana – seafood, shellfish
karanga – call, summon, welcome; formal or ceremonial call
kaumātua – elder/elders
kia ora – greeting
kina – sea urchin
kōauau – small cross blown flute
manawarū – anxious, uneasy; enraptured, ecstatic;
Manawarū – rural community in the Waikato in New Zealand
mihi – greeting
Ōrākau – site of the battle known as 'Rewi's last stand' that took place in 1864
pākehā – New Zealander of European descent
pākehātanga – pākehā culture, pākehā way of life
Papatūānuku – Earth Mother
pāua – shellfish, abalone

poi – light ball on a string twirled rhythmically in song, kapahaka art form

Poi E – number-one hit song released in 1984 by the Patea Māori Club

pop a Mangere – to do a bomb into a river/lake or pool (https://www.youtube.com/watch?v=YUt2VZNbN8o)

pūtōrino – large traditional flute

pūkana – to dilate the eyes; done by both genders when performing haka and waiata to emphasise particular words and to add excitement to the performance.

reo – language

rātā – a native vine

Rewi's last stand – reference to the final battle of the Waikato wars which took place at Ōrākau after the invasion of Waikato by government forces. This was part of the 19th century New Zealand wars, fought in the North Island between the military forces of the colonial government and different federations of Māori tribes.

Taranaki – the region in the west of the North Island in the vicinity of Mount Taranaki

tawa – a tall tree with yellow-green foliage of long, narrow leaves. The bark is smooth and dark brown. Found throughout the North Island and in northern areas of the South Island.

taonga – something precious which may be tangible or intangible

taonga pūoro – singing treasures, traditional Māori musical instruments

Te Urewera – region of New Zealand in the North Island

tī kōuka – cabbage tree

waiata – song, songs

whakapapa – genealogy

whare – house

wharenui – large house, meeting house; main building of marae where guests are accommodated.

Note

I am indebted to Nolan Hodgson as well as the online Māori Dictionary accessed at https://maoridictionary.co.nz for guidance on compiling this glossary.

Acknowledgements

I honour the land of Aotearoa New Zealand and the people I have encountered there in both my professional and personal journeys. My time in New Zealand has been one of growth and challenge in ways I had never imagined and I am warmed by the embrace I carry with me from the land and the karanga that calls across the oceans and holds me as I make a new home in England. I honour my ancestors who stand with me and am reminded of my Grandfather's handwritten pages of stories and poems and tobacco tins of snowdrops posted from Lincolnshire to Hertfordshire carefully unwrapped by my small hands. My mother's poems, received at various milestones in my life, are a reminder that the written word can sometimes carry things the spoken word cannot.

I acknowledge the people whose stories are held in these pages, and the generosity with which they have given consent and approval for their stories to be shared. I have not had to pilot a plane of this shape and size before and my heartfelt thanks go to the therapists (the crew) who have borne with me during false take-offs and bumpy almost-landings (reminiscent of the first time I experienced a 'bunny-hop' and 'go-around' when the plane I was travelling on was unable to land first time at Wellington airport due to high winds!). I am deeply indebted to the writers who have committed their time and energy to the book. I am sustained by the beautiful weekend at Teal Bay, and the ongoing connection and collaboration that has been at the heart of this venture. Thank you to Carolyn Ayson for additional thoughts and references for the introduction. Ali Talmage for support with the grant application to Music Therapy New Zealand, and for coordinating the book launches in New Zealand with Marie Willis and Libby Johns. Kenny Willis for his additional design work on the flyer and invitations.

Thank you to three amazingly talented women: Robina Adamson, Anne Bailey and Stephanie Nierstenhoefer. Your beautiful artwork, eye for detail and belief in the project has been inspirational.

To the amazing Sarah Hoskyns, thank you for taking time out from landing your own 'jumbo jets' to clamber aboard this little plane and add a thoughtful foreword. Your support and encouragement along the way has been invaluable. And to Waireti Roestenburg for insightful consultation on cultural matters, healing waiata and for helping to hold some of my journey along the way.

I thank my colleagues, past and present, in New Zealand and in England for allowing me a little space to indulge a love of poetry and writing and bring this into the workplace from time to time. Thank you to those who have shared that passion and introduced me to new poets and writers along the way. To my psychotherapy and counselling colleagues and mentors in New Zealand; Margot Solomon, Gillian Bowie, Leela Anderson in particular – thank you.

I am grateful to Peta Wellstead and Chris Rutter at Mountain Girl Publishing for their hard work and guidance in getting the book from a series of word documents to what you hold in your hand.

I especially acknowledge Music Therapy New Zealand and the Project Grants Group whose generous grant from the Erika Schloss Fund has made this book possible. Thank you for your confidence in me and in the project.

My friends, Cara Anning and Steph Nierstenhoefer, for always being there and offering strong hands to hold me on this journey. Biz Hayman for reconnecting and Anne Bailey for refuge in the beautiful Bay of Plenty.

Finally, thank you to my family. My husband, Ian, for inspiration, conversation, and sharing discoveries from narrative therapy. My children, Leon, Erin and Rose, for your patience, occasional editing suggestions and technical support.

And thank you to Richard Dalziel for *Only Connect*.

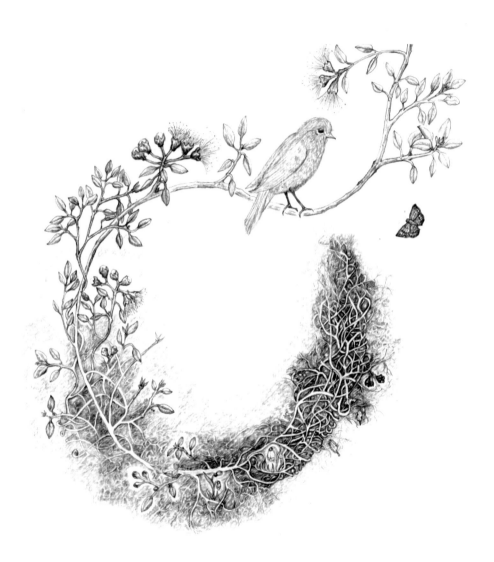